The Juice Lady's

REMEDIES

FOR STRESS & ADRENAL FATIGUE

CHERIE CALBOM, MS, CN

Most CHARISMA HOUSE BOOK GROUP products are available at special quantity discounts for bulk purchase for sales promotions, premiums, fund-raising, and educational needs. For details, write Charisma House Book Group, 600 Rinehart Road, Lake Mary, Florida 32746, or telephone (407) 333-0600.

THE JUICE LADY'S REMEDIES FOR STRESS AND ADRENAL FATIGUE by Cherie Calbom
Published by Siloam
Charisma Media/Charisma House Book Group
600 Rinehart Road
Lake Mary, Florida 32746
www.charismahouse.com

Cover design by Justin Evans
Design Director: Bill Johnson

Visit the author's website at www.juiceladycherie.com.

Library of Congress Cataloging-in-Publication Data:
An application to register this book for cataloging has been submitted to the Library of Congress.
International Standard Book Number: 978-1-62136-567-9
E-book ISBN: 978-1-62136-568-6

While the author has made every effort to provide accurate telephone numbers and Internet addresses at the time of publication, neither the publisher nor the author assumes any responsibility for errors or for changes that occur after publication.

14 15 16 17 18 — 9 8 7 6 5 4 3 2 1

Printed in the United States of America

CONTENTS

Introduction

MY STORY of HOPE and HEALING

S ITTING BY THE window one day in my father's home staring at the snow-topped mountains in the distance, I imagined that people were enjoying the hiking trails and perhaps someone was climbing the mountain that day. It was early June, and the weather was beautiful. I wished I had the strength to just walk around the block. But I was too sick and tired—I could barely walk around the house. I had been sick for a couple of years and just kept getting worse. "Will I ever be well again?" I wondered.

When I turned thirty, I had to quit my job. I had chronic fatigue syndrome and fibromyalgia that made me so sick I couldn't work. I felt as though I had a never-ending flu. Constantly feverish with swollen glands and perennially lethargic, I was also in constant pain. My body ached as though I'd been bounced around in a washing machine.

I had moved back to my father's home in Colorado to try and recover. But not one doctor had an answer as to what I should do to facilitate healing. So I went to some health food stores and browsed around, talked with employees, and read a few books. I decided that everything I'd been doing—such as eating fast food, granola for dinner, and not eating vegetables—was tearing down my health rather than healing my body. I read about juicing and whole foods, and it made sense. So I bought a juicer and designed a program I could follow.

I juiced and ate a nearly perfect diet of live and whole foods for three months. There were ups and downs throughout. I had days where I felt encouraged that I was making some progress but other days when I felt worse. Those were discouraging and made me wonder if health was the elusive dream. No one told me about detox reactions, which was what I was experiencing. I was obviously very toxic, and my body was cleansing away all that stuff that had made me sick. This caused some not-so-good days amid the promising ones.

But one morning I woke up early—early for me, which was around 8:00 a.m.—without an alarm sounding off. I felt like someone had given me a new body in the night. I had so much energy I actually wanted to go jogging. What had happened? This new sensation of health had just appeared with the morning sun. But actually my body had been healing all along; it just had not manifested until that day. What a wonderful sense of being alive! I looked and felt completely renewed.

With my juicer in tow and a new lifestyle fully embraced, I returned to Southern California a couple weeks later to finish writing my first book. For nearly a year it was "ten steps forward" with great health and more energy and stamina than I'd ever remembered. Then, all of a sudden, I took a giant step back.

The Event That Took My Breath Away

July fourth was a beautiful day like so many others in Southern California. I celebrated the holiday with friends that evening at a backyard barbecue. We put on jackets to insulate against the cool evening air and watched fireworks light up the night sky. I returned just before midnight to the house I was sitting for vacationing friends who lived in a lovely neighborhood not far from some family members. I was in bed just a bit after midnight.

I woke up shivering some time later. "Why is it so cold?" I wondered as I rolled over to see the clock; it was 3:00 a.m. That's when I noticed that the door was open to the backyard. "Wonder how that happened?" I thought as I was about to get up to close and lock it. That's when I noticed him crouched in the shadows of the corner of the room—a shirtless young guy in shorts. I blinked twice, trying to deny what I was seeing. Instead of running, he leaped off the floor and ran toward me. He pulled a pipe from his shorts and began attacking me, beating me repeatedly over the head and yelling, "Now you are dead!" We fought, or I should say I tried to defend myself and grab the pipe. It finally flew out of his hands. That's when he choked me to unconsciousness. I felt life leaving my body.

In those last few seconds I knew I was dying. "This is it, the end of my life," I thought. I felt sad for the people who loved me and how they would feel about this tragic event. Then I felt my spirit leave in a sensation of popping out of my body and floating upward. Suddenly everything was peaceful and still. I sensed I was traveling, at what seemed like the speed of light, through black space. I saw what looked like lights twinkling in the distance. But all of a sudden I was back in my body, outside the house, clinging to a fence at the end of the dog run. I don't know how I got there. I screamed for help with all the breath I had. It was my third scream that took all my strength. I felt it would be my last. Each time I screamed, I passed out and landed on the cement. I then had to pull myself up again. But this time a neighbor heard me and sent her husband to help. Within a short time I was on my way to the hospital.

Lying on a cold gurney at 4:30 a.m. chilled to the bone, in and out of consciousness, I tried to assess my injuries, which was virtually impossible. When I finally looked at my right hand, I almost passed out again. My ring finger was barely hanging on by a small piece of skin. My hand was split open, and I could see deep inside. The next thing I knew, I was being wheeled off to surgery. Later I learned that I had suffered serious injuries to my head, neck, back, and right hand, with multiple head wounds and part of my scalp torn from my head. I also incurred numerous cracked teeth that resulted in several root canals and crowns months later.

My right hand sustained the most severe injuries, with two knuckles crushed to mere bone fragments that had to be held together by three metal pins. Six months after the attack I still couldn't use it. The cast I wore—with bands holding up the ring finger, which had almost been torn from my hand, and various odd-shaped molded parts—looked like something from a science-fiction movie. I felt and looked worse than hopeless, with a shaved top of my head, totally red and swollen eyes, a gash on my face, a useless right hand, terrorizing fear, and barely enough energy to get dressed in the morning. I was an emotional wreck. I couldn't sleep at night—not even a minute. It was torturous. Never mind that I was staying with a cousin and his family. There was no need to worry about safety from a practical point of view, but that made no difference emotionally. I'd lie in bed all night and stare at the ceiling or the bedroom door. I had five lights that I kept on all night. I'd try to read, but my eyes would sting. I could sleep for only a little while during the day.

But the worst part was the pain in my soul that nearly took my breath away. All the emotional pain of the attack joined up with the pain and trauma of my past for an emotional tsunami. My past had been riddled with loss, trauma, and anxiety. My brother died when I was two. My mother had died of cancer when I was six. I couldn't remember much about her death—the memories seemed blocked. But my cousin said I fainted at her funeral. That told me the impact was huge.

I lived for the next three years with my maternal grandparents and father. But Grandpa John, the love of my life, died when I was nine—the loss was immeasurable. Four years later my father was involved in a very tragic situation that would take far too long to discuss here, but to sum it up—it was horrific. He was no longer in my daily life. I felt terrified about my future. My grandmother was eighty-six. I had no idea how many more years she would live. The next year I moved to Oregon to live with an aunt and uncle until I graduated from high school.

As you can probably imagine, wrapped in my soul was a huge amount of anguish and pain with all sorts of triggers for emotional and binge eating. I know firsthand about eating-disorder behavior—binge eating and then not eating anything for a few days. I know what it is to get triggered emotionally and be clueless as to what set off an eating binge. Food is immediate comfort. It's often the first thing we turn to. It was for me. But not wanting to gain a lot of weight, I would then avoid food for a day or two after binge eating.

After the attack it took every ounce of my will, faith, and trust in God, deep spiritual work, alternative medical help, extra vitamins and minerals, vegetable juicing, emotional release, healing prayer, and numerous detox programs to heal physically, mentally, and emotionally. I met a nutritionally minded physician who had healed his own slow mending broken bones with lots of vitamin-mineral IVs. He gave me similar IVs. Juicing, cleansing, nutritional supplements, a nearly perfect diet, prayer, and physical therapy helped my bones and other injuries heal.

After following this regimen for about nine months, what my hand surgeon said would be impossible became real—a fully restored, fully functional hand. He had told me I'd never use my right hand again and that it wasn't even possible to put in plastic knuckles because of its poor condition. But my knuckles did indeed re-form primarily through prayer, and function of my hand returned. A day came when he told me I was completely healed, and though he admitted he didn't believe in miracles, he said, "You're the closest thing I've seen to one."

The healing of my hand was indeed a miracle! I had a useful hand again, and my career in writing was not over as I thought it would be. My inner wounds were what seemed severest in the end and the hardest to heal. Nevertheless, they mended too. I experienced healing from the painful memories and trauma of the attack and the wounds from the past through prayer, laying on of hands, and deep emotional healing work. I called them the *kitchen angels*—the ladies who prayed for me around their kitchen table week after week until my soul was healed. I cried endless buckets of tears that had been pent up in my soul. It all needed release. Forgiveness and letting go came in stages and was an integral part of my total healing. I had to be honest about what I really felt and willing to face the pain and toxic emotions confined inside, and then let them go. Finally, one day after a long journey—I felt free. A time came when I could celebrate the Fourth of July without fear.

Today I know more peace and health than I ever thought would be possible. I have experienced what it is to feel whole—complete; not damaged, broken, wounded, or impaired; but truly healed and restored in body, soul, and spirit. And I'm not plagued with emotional eating anymore.

When I look back to that first day in the hospital after many hours of surgery, it's amazing to me that I made it. My hand was resting in a sling hanging above my head. It was wrapped with so much stuff it looked like George Foreman's boxing glove. My face was black and blue and my eyes were red—no whites—they were completely red. A maintenance man came into my room for a repair and did a double take. He asked if I'd been hit by a truck! I felt like I had. As I lay there alone with tears streaming down my face, I asked God if He could bring something good out of this horrific situation. I needed something to hang onto. My prayer was answered. Eventually I knew my purpose was to love people to life through my writing and nutritional information to help them find their way to health and healing. If I could recover from all that had happened to me, they could too. No matter what anyone faced, there was hope.

I want you to know that you are loved, and I send you my love between the lines of this book and with the juice and raw food recipes. There is hope for you. You do not have to continue suffering the results of stress and exhaustion. No matter what challenges you face, there are answers that will heal your body, mind, and spirit. There's a purpose for your life, just as there was for mine. You need to be strong and well to complete your purpose. You can be greatly served by a positive mind and an optimistic attitude. To that end I have specially designed *The Juice Lady's Remedies for Stress and Adrenal Fatigue* just for you. With God's help and the latest nutritional data in this book, you can facilitate abundant health and learn the right way to live your life to the fullest and finish well.

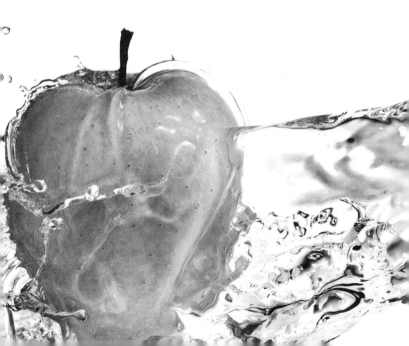

Chapter 1

STRESS and FOOD

FROM INFANCY WE have developed deep feelings around food, often buried in the subconscious. When we cried as babies, we were fed; the distress caused by hunger was replaced with a warm, full tummy. As children, food soothed our tears and calmed our fears. As adults, we self-medicate our anxieties, hurts, fears, loneliness, and disappointments. We stuff down emotions with our favorite comfort foods. Food is a reliable friend—consistent and dependable. It can be a surrogate for human contact and the bridge by which we form connections.

How many parties or social gatherings have you been to that didn't serve food? Food is the center of celebrations. Think about Thanksgiving, Christmas, Hanukkah, birthdays, the Fourth of July, weddings, dating, and business parties. I'll bet you have a long list of "celebration foods" you enjoy at such times. We all have positive emotions regarding our favorite foods served on special occasions. Most of us also have a list of comfort foods that we turn to when we're unhappy, sad, stressed out, angry, or experiencing any number of other emotions. When the going gets tough, we often gravitate to the feel-good foods we remember from our youth—everything from macaroni and cheese to mashed potatoes and gravy, hot bread and butter, chocolate chip cookies (did you eat the dough?), candy, or ice cream.

If your boyfriend dumps you, grilled fish and steamed asparagus probably won't cut it. If you get fired from your job, I'll bet vegetable soup and salad are not what you'll order for lunch. What do you eat when bad things happen? What do you reach for when you're all stressed out? If you're like most people, you are going to go for foods that are emotionally comforting. And those are usually the fare that's on the "off limits" list.

Many of us have grown up on brand-name products that have little in common with the whole foods from which they were processed. Many times we prefer these foods in times of stress. Even for those who have eaten a whole-foods diet for years, there's still, somewhere back in the recesses of our soul, fond memories of such things as steaming bowls of canned chicken noodle soup served with a sandwich made of soft, snowy white bread grilled in margarine and stuffed with melted, orange-colored cheese. Mothers, who were either frazzled by overwork or seduced by the concept of convenience, served high-carb processed foods to us with love, and although they may have been anything but wholesome, in our subconscious mind they're still desirable and take us back to the comfort of home.

But what is the price of unhealthy comfort foods or simple-pleasure indulgences? Many of us could say weight gain for one, poor health for another. Unfortunately, all of us who grew up on a diet of brand-name fare and sugar-laden, refined-carb foods have some major rethinking and attitude adjustments to do if we want to successfully adopt a healthy lifestyle that will promote long-term adrenal strength, weight management, and vibrant health.

We've also grown up with the "bigger is better" mentality in America. It's the "super-size me" idea that's become so popular today in everything from all-you-can-eat buffets to Big Macs and colossal shakes. Have you seen the movie *Super-Size Me* (2004)? Morgan Spurlock, the film director and subject of the movie, ruins his health in short order eating super-sized, fast-food meals at McDonald's. He cut the project short because of the alarming decline in his blood work and symptoms of poor health.

We've come to believe we don't get our money's worth unless we're served a large portion. So when we're dealing with emotional eating or cravings, we not only want our favorite indulgences, but we also want it in large quantity. Herein lie two challenges—the "off limits" food and the quantity that we eat.

What Triggers Stress Eating?

The stuff that can trigger a flood of emotions is limitless. Maybe it's a bill you can't pay, a stressful day at work, arguing with a family member, or getting stood up by a date. When a flood of emotional energy comes pouring down your psychological pipes, more often than not the reaction is to run to the fridge for your favorite food and suppress the whole thing.

At such times you eat food not because you're hungry but because you're sad, depressed, discouraged, bored, or anxious. That "little devil" on your shoulder says, "Yep, you're right! It's been a really crummy day, and you deserve this. Go ahead. Eat a heaping bowl of ice cream or a large piece of double-chocolate cheesecake. You'll feel a whole lot better!"

Stress of any kind triggers a drop in serotonin levels, which can cause cravings for sweets and starches such as cookies, pasta, or bread. Women are usually more susceptible to stress eating because of fluctuating hormones. PMS can cause women to eat junk food and sweets.

Momentarily these foods can help improve mood and encourage happy memories or feelings. (But *momentarily* is the key word.) Their lure has both chemical and emotional triggers. Some foods work on serotonin levels in the brain, producing a calming effect because they produce higher levels of serotonin, which is a little like "instant Prozac." Others work on an emotional level, reminding us of comfort and warmth. But the effects don't last, and we're often worse off than before we started eating the junk.

Emotions have roots in the past. You may not be able to consciously spot the trigger that sends you running to the cupboard or grocery store, but it's there in your subconscious. You may hear a familiar old song playing on the radio as you drive home from work. It just happens that it was your song when you and your high school sweetheart were in love. Then he dropped you for another girl, and you drowned your sorrows in chocolate chip cookies. All of a sudden you have an insatiable desire to eat chocolate when you hear the song, even though it's been years since you've thought of that guy. You probably don't think about him when you hear the song; you just want chocolate!

Your mother's admonition "Don't spoil your dinner!" just flew straight out the window. Whatever happens in your moments of binge eating, don't be too hard on yourself. Most of the patterns you're working hard to overcome started when you were young. You might not remember where or when they started, but they're there nevertheless. Your earliest memories often revolve around food—calorie-rich, nutrient-light fare.

Fear, pain, sorrow, joy, and happiness—almost always these emotions are associated with the really bad stuff: sugar, white flour, and salty snacks. But don't give up. You can change this pattern. If your brain can grow new dendrites and your liver can rejuvenate itself, you can develop new patterns of eating and behaving.

Addicted to an Adrenaline Rush?

Some people look for the excitement of misery, chaos, or crisis. It's the "drug of choice." They like pushing the envelope, going to the edge, seeing how far they can take things. Not surprisingly many of these people grew up in crazy, dysfunctional households with problem parents or siblings or with chaos, trauma, abuse, loss, or crisis as a familiar scenario in childhood. They don't know how to function unless things are in turmoil, and they almost panic when things are going well. Have you ever thought that this might be a scenario you experience?

When we think about all the challenging things that have happened in our past, we know we don't want the future to be a repeat. But on a subconscious level we may be creating repeats over and over again.

Psychologists tell us that we can get addicted to the highs and lows of hormone rushes produced by trauma, tragedy, crises, or chaos. Some people are *drama queens*; other people like to stir things up. Some people seem to find themselves in messes over and over again. Other people have to make sure something goes wrong, even when everything is going well. These people are addicted to chaos or crisis.

Shots of adrenaline and cortisol pump through our bodies at these times and take us back to early days when those hormones pumped through our system like little torpedoes. Though it's not pleasant, we can crave it—become addicted to it. We somehow seek to bring all this familiar emotional and hormonal chaos back. It trashes our bodies, but we can't see the damage. We just feel the familiar rush. Often food is tied in with this whole scenario. It may be what we ate during those crisis times that we crave when crisis hits in the present. Indeed, food affects our biochemistry. Many foods and substances can help us achieve those highs and chaotic hormone rushes.

You can overcome food addictions, binge eating, and emotional eating. I've overcome them. Many other people have overcome them. Angela Stokes tells her story in *Raw Emotions* of how her overeating caused her to reach a weight of 300 pounds. She learned how to overcome emotional eating, cravings, and food addictions and lost over 160 pounds. She's taken her life back while actively inspiring others to do the same!

In this next chapter I will show you practical ways to lower your stress levels and combat triggers that cause you to stress eat.

Chapter 2

YOU CAN'T CONTROL EVERYTHING

WHEN THE TOILET overflows, the car breaks down, or your computer crashes, you certainly can't know how to fix everything. We think we can manage the universe, but we aren't experts on all fronts. We just can't control it all. When stuff happens, our emotions often spin out of control. That's when we run for our favorite comfort food. For me it used to be mashed potatoes with a boatload of butter. I even started buying boxes of instant mashed potatoes years ago so that I could make them quickly. (Take heart; there's hope. I haven't bought those in years.) Whatever we eat doesn't solve the problem, as you know, and often makes it worse. Meantime the problem's still there.

The computer guy probably never wants to eat a bag of chips out of frustration when he's working on a computer problem. But when my computer crashes or my Internet connection goes down, I feel helpless and hopeless. What makes you feel helpless and out of control?

While I was working on this chapter, my furnace went down. It was cold outside. I didn't want to call the furnace company. It costs sixty-five dollars for them to walk through my front door and tell me that the panels to my furnace don't fit properly, and therefore the little white button is not getting pushed in to turn the furnace on. I face this challenge nearly every time I change the filter in my furnace. I know the panels don't fit right. It's tricky to get them on. Today it didn't work no matter what I did. But I'm juice fasting today. Just consuming fresh veggie juices and raw soup. I'm not going to break my juice fast simply because I'm frustrated. So I did the one thing that works. It works every single time. I've tried all the clever little suggestions that experts write about that are supposed to help us get through these emotionally upsetting events. None of them have worked for me. But this works.

Prayer. That's right. Prayer. When I can't figure it out, I've learned to pray. So I just simply prayed for a furnace angel to come and help me with a creative idea. Sure enough, I got an idea. Duct tape. (My fix-it angel loves duct tape.) A few strips of duct tape wadded up and stuck in just the right spot of the door panel, and *voilà*! The furnace was humming. A few years ago I'd have been a wreck, smacking the door panel, freezing, and emotionally tied in a knot. I'd probably have eaten a lot more than a bowl of instant mashed potatoes with butter.

But now my problem was solved. I was happy and at peace. I grabbed my big glass of beet, carrot, cucumber, kale, lemon, and ginger juice and sat down to drink my lunch.

Try it! Whether you're sitting at the genius bar waiting for a computer geek to fix your crashed computer and hopefully retrieve all the files you're fearing are permanently lost, or you're sitting on hold waiting for your high-speed Internet server rep to figure out why you can't connect—pray. Pray for the person working on your problem. Pray for creative ideas for the fix-it person. Pray for yourself and your peace of mind. It's amazing what happens. It can change your entire life.

You can't control everything that happens. You can control your reactions. And you can let go and pray.

Admit, Acknowledge, Confront

You may not have thought a lot about the binge eating you do from time to time. These episodes just happen, right? And life goes on. But life doesn't go on well, and the binges will never change—you'll never change—until you admit that you binge and confront your behavior.

I've written more than twenty-one books, taught numerous classes, and spoken to large groups of people at seminars. People take notes, underline points in my books, and talk a lot about eating the right foods. It's usually emotional eating and binge eating that keep them from the weight they want and the good health they long for.

If you're keeping your binge eating a secret, maybe not even admitting it to yourself, you will stay on that emotional-eating roller coaster for a long time. Isn't it time to take a good look at what's going on? How is your mind influencing you? How is your past triggering you? You may be trying to hold that emotional beach ball under water with all your might, but every once in a while the thing just pops up. The volcano of past experiences with the emotions they spawned is buried in your subconscious. These emotions erupt every now and then.

Your story might tear my heart in two. A lot of people who suffer with binge eating, emotional eating, or more serious eating disorders have suffered abuse, deprivation, painful loss, or rejection in their past. Heartbreaking things can happen to us. Life can offer us a rough road to travel. But at some point we have to ask ourselves if we're going to allow what happened in the past to wreck our present and future.

While you can't control what happened to you, you can control your response to what happened then and your response to what happens now and in the future. No matter how many times you have tried and failed to choose a healthy lifestyle, don't lose hope. You can do this. It just takes a willing heart. You have that. That's why you chose this book. You were looking for hope and a plan that would work. Willpower or gutting it out works only so long. Then the whole thing snaps like a broken rubber band. And you're right back to your old behavior. But a willing heart that's open to change and to finding a new way of responding to life—well, that kind of humble approach gets you further than you'd think. A willing heart looks for creative ways and helping angels to get you through the tough moments of life. I promise, you can get through those moments of your life, and you can change.

Mindful Eating

A study done by Duke and Indiana State University found that mindfulness, including specific instructions to slowly savor the flavor of food and be aware of how much food is enough, helped to reduce eating binges from an average of four binges per week to one.[1]

It's rarely easy to make a major change, even when our better sense says this is the best program and the path to fitness. No matter how convinced or motivated we are, there's still a little voice somewhere in our inner depths screaming, "I want sugar-frosted breakfast flakes!" Or whatever was a favorite. And regardless of what foods we choose as a temporary "fix" for our screaming emotions, the positive effects are only momentary. In the end they set us up for real depression about our weight gain, low energy, or ill health. It's not always easy to make changes, but if we consider that making no change can mean a lifetime of stressed adrenals, illness, and fatigue, the decision to change becomes compelling.

When an emotional binge strikes, you might want to think about dealing with yourself just as you would a small child who picks up something that could be harmful. Most of us would quickly find something to give the child in exchange for the harmful object so we could then easily take away the thing that could harm him. Start working with yourself in this way. There's an inner child inside of you. Just grabbing the coveted "off limits" food or drink out of your grasp isn't going to work for long. Rebellion will pop up and send you overboard.

So rather than trying to force on yourself a strict rule of life, develop your list of exchanges for these moments of cravings. Say you want a cookie. What substitute can you offer yourself that's actually good for you? It might be a dehydrated cracker that has the texture of a cookie.

It might be a piece of fruit or something with the fiber inulin, which has a sweet taste. You can say to your inner self, "We can't have that, but we can have this." What can you do when you want ice cream? You can make recipes for frozen desserts that are just fruit you freeze and blend up. I've developed a recipe with veggies—the "Icy, Spicy Gazpacho." It's slushy, spicy, and works for me. You could also freeze coconut water and blend that up. It makes a delicious slush.

Finding Solutions

Ask yourself the following questions when you're tempted to emotionally eat or go on food binges:

- What am I really feeling?
- Can I just be with this feeling?
- If I eat this fattening food or go on a sugar binge, what will it cost me in the long run?
- What's really important to me now?
- What do I want to achieve?
- Is there a better way to take care of myself both emotionally and physically?
- What can I give myself right now that won't cost me my power?
- How can I nurture myself right now without hurting myself?
- If I were a child, how would I like to be comforted?
- What can I do today that will make me feel good tomorrow?

- How can I reward myself with things that are good for me?

Develop a List of Healthy Substitutes and Rewards

Make a list of healthy food substitutes and keep the foods on hand. What nonfood rewards can you think of that are good for you? Following are a few suggestions:

- Call a friend.

- Take a walk.

- Watch a favorite movie.

- Take a hot bath by candlelight with your favorite music and a cup of herbal tea.

- Work out and work away your worries; exercise can help—it raises endorphins and other "feel-good" hormones.

A Plan of Action

Get a journal and write about your food cravings. Writing about cravings can be helpful to identify emotions that cause the cravings. Try to identify a pattern as to what triggers them.

- Let your emotions speak rather than suppressing them; write about them.

- Ask your cravings questions. You may be surprised at what you hear. The point is to hear them out and find out what your real need is.

- Food suppresses emotions; allow your feelings and emotions to be heard and understood.

- Think about a trim, healthy person you admire. How do you think that person would handle a food-binge urge?

- Learn to have fun without food.

- Cultivate personal power.

- Increase nurturing life experiences that can help you get beyond junk food and comfort food eating.

- Accept your emotions rather than stuffing them or shutting them down.

- Allow your emotions to come up and let them go.

- Courageously face painful situations and emotions without stuffing them or covering them up.

- Invite nurturing people into your life.

- Cultivate self-loving experiences.

- Practice stress reduction.

Seven Steps You Can Take to Overcome Stress Eating

Get a plan clearly in mind about what you're going to do the next time you're tempted to eat the foods you know aren't on your healthy diet plan.

Associate your actions with the outcome of your choices. Be as graphic as you can and try to actually feel what you would experience physically if you ate the things that you shouldn't eat. Or if you experience no adverse physical sensations, think about how this food might impact your health.

Picture the foods that are detrimental to your health with a very negative symbol, such as the words "rat poison" written above them, or any other negative association that will really turn you off.

Associate the foods that are part of your health program with positive thoughts such as, "Mineral water with a slice of lemon is a great party drink! It's better for me than alcohol, and it tastes great!"

Develop a list of "right choice" comfort foods that you can turn to when you're emotionally down. Write down a list of acceptable foods for celebrations. Make sure you have some of these foods on hand at all times so you aren't tempted to go out for ice cream or nachos when your emotions are screaming for comfort, when you are anxious and want to stuff the whole thing, or when you feel like celebrating.

The next time you go out to dinner or prepare a special meal at home, and you're tempted to throw caution to the wind and splurge, remember that what you eat will impact your health. Think about how you will feel the next morning when you wake up with a headache and you reflect on what you did. You've embarked on a special mission to restore your adrenals to health, get fit, and improve your overall well-being.

If you splurge, don't punish yourself. Start over the very next meal with a positive plan to make wise choices in the future. And no matter what, never succumb to the temptation of throwing the whole plan out because you've blown it a time or two. Just pick yourself up and get back in the race!

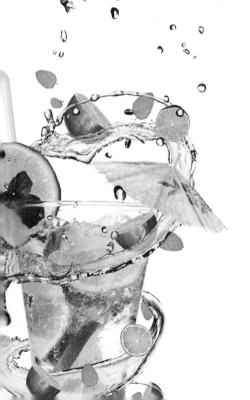

Chapter 3

CHRONIC STRESS and ADRENAL FATIGUE

ADRENAL FATIGUE IS a collection of symptoms that results when the adrenal glands do not function at their optimal level. The fatigue is not relieved by sleep. As a result, changes may occur in carbohydrate, protein, and fat metabolism; blood sugar balance; energy production; fluid and electrolyte balance; cardiovascular function; sleep patterns; mood; menstrual and menopausal symptoms; and even sex drive. People whose adrenals are fatigued often have to use coffee, colas, or other stimulants to get going in the morning and to prop themselves up during the day.

Adrenal fatigue often develops over a period of years due to unhealthy lifestyle factors such as poor eating habits, poor sleep patterns, and/or chronic stress. For example, someone who eats refined foods and sugar will have an imbalance in the hormones insulin and cortisol. Eating poorly can, over time, lead to insulin resistance and eventually diabetes, which usually takes years to develop. The constant secretion of cortisol in response to eating poorly and/or dealing with chronic stress can weaken the adrenal glands and eventually lead to adrenal fatigue.

Similarly, not getting enough sleep can weaken the adrenals. Many people stay up late watching television, surfing the Internet, staying out with friends, or studying. They get only five to seven hours of sleep; some even less. This is not enough. Most people need eight to nine hours of sleep. An occasional short night of sleep is not a big problem, but on a regular basis it can affect cortisol levels and weaken adrenal glands. And not dealing with stress effectively has a similar effect on the adrenal and thyroid glands, weakening both.

Trauma, which can be either physical or emotional in nature, such as a car accident, the death of a loved one, a divorce, or loss of a job, can trigger this disorder as well. This doesn't mean that such traumas cause the immediate development of adrenal fatigue, but they can be the trigger that over time leads to its development.

When the adrenal glands are weakened, it puts the body in a state of catabolism—the body begins breaking down. When the body is in a catabolic state, the thyroid gland will slow down (become hypothyroid) in an attempt to conserve energy and prevent the body from breaking down more. This makes sense in that hypothyroidism slows down the metabolism.

There is no magic bullet or supplement that can quickly cure these conditions. But by changing your lifestyle, you can heal these glands and restore your health. It usually doesn't take too long before you start feeling better, and symptoms should lessen within a few weeks if you strictly adhere to my living foods and juice program. It will take time, though, to completely heal. It's very important to remember that when you start feeling a little better, you should not abandon your healthy lifestyle program and go back to your former favorite foods.

Adrenal Fatigue Followed My Attack

If you read the introduction, you know that I was attacked in the night by a burglar while I was house-sitting for friends. Following the attack, I suffered extreme adrenal fatigue. I was so tired I could barely drag myself through a day. It felt like I had a ball and chain wrapped around my waist.

Just getting dressed in the morning was a huge effort. I remember sitting on the floor in the corner of my bedroom thinking that I was so tired I couldn't get up off the floor. Life was so painful and difficult that it didn't seem worth it to go on. I remember thinking I could go deep inside my soul where there was peace and hide. But I recalled something about a catatonic state (one of near unconsciousness often brought on by shock) from psychology 101. My professor had mentioned that it was hard to bring people out of that state. I thought I'd better not go there just in case I would not want to be there someday. I decided to hang on for just one more day, albeit by a thin thread of hope that things might improve. Obviously they did.

I looked at my picture on my website the other day. It didn't seem possible that the glowing person I was looking at was the same person who once sat in a corner of a room one thought away from "checking out" for good.

Healing the adrenals, indeed the entire body, takes work. It takes the best nutrition you can possibly eat and drink, with plenty of live foods rich in biophotons that give life to your body. It takes nutritional supplements of superior quality. It may take a few IVs of Meyer's Cocktail (vitamin C drip with other nutrients), which is what I got, along with prayer and intense emotional work.

Factors That Put Excess Stress on the Adrenals

- Bitterness, anger, fear, anxiety, guilt, depression, and other negative emotions
- Physical or mental strain, overwork, driven
- Excessive exercise
- Sleep deprivation
- Staying up late even though tired
- Light-cycle disruption (night shift work or often going to sleep late)
- Surgery, trauma, injury, shock, loss, or disappointment
- Chronic inflammation, infection, illness, or pain
- Temperature extremes
- Exposure to toxins
- Nutritional deficiencies
- Severe allergies
- Poor food choices (white flour, low fiber, sugar, too few vegetables and fruit, lack of raw food)
- Using sweet or salty food and sweetened or caffeinated drinks as stimulants when tired

- Feeling or acting powerless
- Continually driving yourself
- Striving to be perfect
- Staying in double binds—no-win situations
- Too few enjoyable and rejuvenating activities

Do You Have Adrenal Fatigue?

Below are symptoms of adrenal fatigue and lifestyle factors that contribute to it to help in determining if this may be a health concern for you.

Symptoms of adrenal fatigue

- Extremely tired, especially in the morning
- Have trouble getting up, even when you've had enough sleep
- Find it difficult to obtain quality sleep; high nighttime cortisol affects REM
- Crave sweets or alcohol
- Salt cravings
- Feel stressed out most of the time
- Feel rundown or overwhelmed
- Have trouble bouncing back from an illness or stressful situation
- Decreased sex drive

- Feel more awake, alert, and energetic after 6:00 p.m. than you do all day
- Asthma, bronchitis, or chronic cough
- Excessive thirst and urination
- Allergies; as adrenal function decreases, allergies worsen
- Recurring infections
- Muscle weakness and back pain
- Dizziness
- Inflammation
- Hypoglycemia
- Headaches
- Hollow cheeks
- Lines in fingertips
- Pale lips
- Balding legs and/or arms
- Behavior or memory problems
- Swelling
- Hemorrhoids
- Varicose veins
- Indigestion
- Hyperpigmentation

IS ADRENAL FATIGUE THE SAME AS CHRONIC FATIGUE SYNDROME?

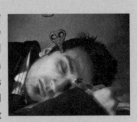

Chronic fatigue syndrome (CFS) and adrenal fatigue are not the same, but adrenal function may play some role in its course. The cause of CFS is unknown, but it is characterized by severe, chronic fatigue of six months or longer that is not attributable to other known medical conditions. It is typically accompanied by some combination of four or more other symptoms that have also lasted for six months or more and are unique to the period of fatigue. These symptoms can include impaired short-term memory or concentration, sore throat, tender lymph nodes, muscle pain, multi-joint pain without swelling or redness, headaches, sleep that is not refreshing, and prolonged malaise after exercise.

A period of physical or emotional stress commonly precedes the onset of CFS. However, people with CFS have been found to produce lower levels of the adrenal stress hormone, cortisol, than do healthy people. Although low cortisol does not seem to cause CFS, and raising cortisol levels does not eliminate it, adrenal fatigue, and its concomitant low production of cortisol and a number of other regulatory hormones, may help predispose a person to its onset or exacerbate the symptoms.

When there is a longer than normal recovery period from CFS, with decreased stamina and pronounced morning tiredness, adrenal fatigue is likely contributing to the symptom picture, no matter the cause of the illness. Providing adequate support for healthy adrenal function can be an important contributing factor in facilitating full recovery from CFS and the maintenance of health and vitality.[1]

What You Can Do to Restore Your Adrenals

- *Reduce stressors.* This is an important step. Emotional stressors such as marital, family, friends, or financial problems need to be dealt with and responded to in a healthy way. Stress causes the adrenal glands to produce more cortisol, which deposits weight on the belly. When the adrenal glands become exhausted, however, they produce less and less cortisol.

- *Sleep.* Rest and sleep are extremely important to heal the adrenals. Get eight to nine hours of sleep or more. Also rest after meals and at midmorning and midafternoon if possible. Adrenal fatigue is a common cause of insomnia. There are two types of insomnia: adrenal hyper function (inability to fall asleep) and adrenal fatigue (inability to stay asleep). If you have hyper-adrenal function, you may have higher than normal levels of cortisol at bedtime so you can't fall asleep. If you can't stay asleep, you may have very low levels of cortisol and may be getting too much neurotransmitter stimulation. As blood sugar levels start to drop during the middle of the night, normally your adrenal glands are secreting cortisol to help push your blood sugar levels back up. That is normal and is what's supposed to happen. If your glands cannot produce enough cortisol to keep your blood sugar levels balanced, you will shift to a backup system that involves the release of epinephrine and norepinephrine. These hormones are central nervous system stimulants that will wake you up. This is why you may seem to be wide-awake with a racing mind around the same time every night, such as 2:00, 3:00, or 4:00 a.m. Sleep medications are not the answer. They have many side effects and don't cure the problem. You can help balance your brain neurotransmitters, with the amino acid program. You can take the free self quiz at www.neurogistics.com. Use my practitioner code SLEEP (all caps.)

- *Gentle exercise* is beneficial, but vigorous exercise depletes the adrenals. Deep breathing and stretching are very beneficial.

- *Detoxification.* Using an infrared sauna will greatly speed up recovery. If you are in adrenal burnout, use the sauna daily for no more than thirty minutes. Once or twice a week is excellent for maintenance.

- Go to bed by 10:00 p.m.

- Don't use white, processed salt. Use only Celtic or gray sea salt or pink Himalayan salt. The adrenals need good salt. Use sea salt to taste in your dishes and your adrenals will thank you!

- Avoid coffee completely.

- Eat no sweets.

- Avoid grains and starches.

- Drink two to three glasses of green veggie juice per day.

- Focus on loving thoughts and activities. What brings you pleasure: being with people you love, enjoying your favorite pets, savoring a delicious meal, taking a relaxing vacation? Such activities short-circuit the harm done by the body's physiological reaction to stress. As my psychotherapist husband says, "Learn to think with your heart." If you learn to regularly experience joy and fulfillment, you will evoke biochemical changes in your body over time that will recharge your adrenals. (My husband recommends the training programs and books from The Institute of HeartMath where he was trained in HeartMath.) Make sure you laugh often and take on fewer activities that feel like obligations. Spend more time with people who make you feel good and less with people who are draining. Have fun.[2]

Supplements for Rebuilding Adrenals

DHEA helps to neutralize cortisol's immune-suppressant effect. It keeps LDL cholesterol levels under control, provides vitality and energy, sharpens the mind, and helps maintain normal sleep patterns. Like norepinephrine and cortisol, DHEA also improves your ability to recover from episodes of stress and trauma, overwork, and temperature extremes. A decline in libido due to falling testosterone levels is often due to declining DHEA levels. This is the root of the testosterone deficiency since DHEA is the main ingredient the body uses to manufacture testosterone. If your adrenals test low, take small doses of pharmaceutical grade DHEA (5–10 mg/day and up to 25 mg once or twice a day. Seek the advice of your health professional.)

Vitamin C needs to increase with adrenal stress. Take between 2,000 and 4,000 mg a day.

Licorice root contains plant hormones that mimic the effects of cortisol. Use licorice root solid extract and start with one-quarter teaspoon three times a day.

Siberian ginseng is related to a precursor for DHEA and cortisol. Take a 100 mg capsule two times a day. However, if it interferes with your sleep, take it before 3:00 p.m.

Get natural sunlight. This is not only good for your adrenal glands, but it also boosts vitamin D. Sunbathe only in the early morning or late afternoon.[3]

You Can be Restored

If you are fatigued and sense you may have low adrenal function, you may want to take the Adrenal Saliva Test. You can order the test from Neurogenics. Just go to www.Neurogistics.com and click "Get Started." Use the practitioner code SLEEP (all caps). You'll be given a customized protocol with guidelines for the right amino acids and supplements for you to take to help correct your imbalances. Or you can call 866-843-8935 for more information.

You can restore burned-out adrenals that are so exhausted they're barely producing cortisol. You can heal your body that feels too tired to move. I know you can. If I could do it, so can you. We're not all that different, you and I. So go for it! Put some of the advice and resources in this book to the test, and give it all you have. One day, my friend, you'll be standing in your dream as well, just as I'm standing in mine.

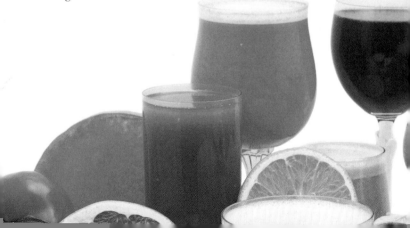

Chapter 4

LIVING FOODS INCREASE VITALITY and INNER PEACE

L IVING FOODS ARE a great weapon against unhealthy cravings during times of high stress. Unlike those prepackaged, nutrient-depleted snacks, living foods "love you back" by giving you a plethora of life-giving nutrients. That equates to higher energy levels, weight loss, detoxification, mental clarity, increased vitality, calmness, and inner peace. Eating a wide variety of produce gives you a powerhouse of vitamins, minerals, enzymes, phytonutrients, and biophotons. Raw foods, which are rich in antioxidants, also help the body remove toxins, thus helping to keep you from getting ill.

A diet that is made up of 60 to 80 percent raw foods is a live foods diet, because the majority of the foods are eaten in their natural state. Eating living foods, especially vegetables, sprouts, wild greens, fruits, nuts, and seeds, is the healthiest for the human body. Truly they can transform you from the inside out.

Raw juices and living foods are packed with a cornucopia of nutrients, including biophotons—those light rays of energy the plants get from the sun. When we cook food, those beautiful rays of energy are destroyed or shrink way down. Professor Fritz-Albert Popp and Dr. H. Niggli are two researchers who have found that the light energy in biophotons is an important aspect of food. The more *light* a food is able to store, the more beneficial the food is to your body. Naturally grown fruits and vegetables that are ripened in the sun are strong sources of light energy. Numerous minute particles of light—biophotons, the smallest units of light—make their way into our cells when we eat these foods. They provide our bodies with important information, and they control complex processes such as ordering and regulating our cells.[1]

Biophotons help to fix errors that have taken place within the body,[2] causing you to start feeling better, lighter, and more energized as time goes on. Your sleep improves, and you may need less of it. Your mind becomes more alert and creative. No longer will you find yourself in a disorganized fog because biophotons help your mind and body to come alive. You will experience more mental energy, and your creativity improves as well because of the electrical stimulation of the biophotons. (Could this be the reboot for dementia or early Alzheimer's disease?) Your metabolism also ramps up, and you burn more calories, helping you get fit with greater ease. In the process your overall health improves. Symptoms of poor health, ailments, and chronic diseases begin to heal. Your whole life changes!

How Living Foods Love You Back

- *Alkalinity.* Most Americans are slightly acidic because most of the American diet (animal products, grains, sugar and sweets of all kinds, coffee, black tea, sodas, sports drinks, and junk food) is acidic or turns acidic when it's digested. This causes a host of problems from weight gain to joint pain. The body tends to store acid in fat cells to protect delicate organs and tissues. It will hold on to fat cells; it will even make more fat cells to protect you. But a living foods diet, which is dominated with fresh vegetables, vegetable juices, fruit, sprouts, seeds, and nuts, provides an abundance of alkalinity. This neutralizes the acids, and the body can let go of fat cells. Many people report that their body also got rid of pain—all sorts of pain throughout the body—when they began juicing and eating a living foods diet.

- *Hydration.* One of the things lost when you cook food is the water content. Our bodies are about 70 percent water. Live foods contain plenty of water. Approximately 85 percent of many fruits and vegetables is water, so eating raw fresh produce is a wonderful way to obtain water. Plenty of water in our system equates to enzymes being able to carry out their metabolic work, and the easier it is for vitamins and minerals to be assimilated into our cells. The more live energy the water holds in the form of biophotons, the better the individual cells function and the higher the quality of your health.

- *Superior protein.* Though not a complete protein, raw plants offer quality amino acids. Cooking denatures the proteins in our food—they coagulate, making them difficult to assimilate. The heat disorganizes their structure, leading to deficiencies of some of the essential amino acids, whereas eating live foods offers amino acids in their best state.

- *Abundant vitamins.* Many vitamins are destroyed when food is cooked or processed.

- *Biophotons.* Plants release biophotons, which can only be measured by special equipment developed by German researchers.[3] These light rays of energy that plants take in from the sun energize our bodies and help our cells communicate more efficiently. Heat and processing destroy them.

- *Greater strength, energy, and stamina.* Dr. Karl Elmer experimented with a raw food diet for top athletes in Germany. He saw improvement in their performance when they changed to an entirely raw food diet.[4] After eating raw food, rather than feeling fatigued or sleepy, most people feel energized. Also, most people eating a high raw food diet experience a more restful sleep and require less of it.

- *Better mental performance.* Your memory and concentration should be clearer. You should be more alert, more creative, and think more logically.

- *Improved digestion due to more enzymes.* Enzymes are important because they are the catalysts of nearly every chemical reaction in our bodies. Vitamins and hormones need enzymes to do optimal work. Live foods contain a good mix of food enzymes. But when food is heated above 118 degrees, enzymes are destroyed, which forces our digestive system to work harder than it should. This can result in partially digested fats, proteins, and starches. When our diet is rich in enzymes, it spares our enzyme-producing organs extra work. That equates to better digestion and more energy.

- *Reduced risk of disease.* A diet rich in raw vegetables and fruit has been shown to lower your risk of cancer and other diseases. Also, according to a study published in the *British Medical Journal*, eating fresh produce on a daily basis has been shown to reduce your chance of death from heart attacks and related problems by as much as 24 percent.[5]

How to Shop for Living Foods

1. Choose real, whole food.

These are the foods that are closest to their natural form and, therefore, retain the most nutrient value and deliver the highest health benefits. They are picked after they've ripened, and they are rich in flavor. They retain natural diversity of taste. They have full nutrient and antioxidant content. And if they are organically grown, seasonal, and local foods, they are the healthiest choices possible.

LIGHT AFFECTS NUTRIENTS

Do you select your produce from the front of a display, or do you reach to the back, hoping you'll find the ones that are freshest and least picked over?

If you think the hidden produce is the best, a new 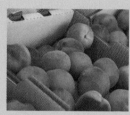 study may convince you to choose your fruits and veggies differently. Scientists from the US Department of Agriculture (USDA) recommend that consumers select their produce from those receiving the greatest light— usually the ones found at the front or top of the display. For example, researchers found that spinach exposed to continuous light during storage was more nutritionally dense than spinach that was continually in the dark. The scientists said light affects the leaves' photosynthetic system, which resulted in an increase in vitamins C, E, K, and folate.[6]

2. Opt for the freshest fruit, vegetables, and legumes you can find.

Choose food items that have been grown organically to avoid toxic pesticides and to get increased nutrition. Buy from local growers whenever possible, because that produce is fresher than anything trucked in from other locations.

3. Choose organic produce.

Organic produce doesn't have the many pesticides known or suspected to cause brain and nervous system damage, cancer, disruption of the endocrine and immune systems, and a host of other toxic effects resulting from pesticides that are in our food supply. Studies have also shown that the organic produce completely surpasses conventional produce in nutritional content.[7] When choosing organically grown foods, look for labels that are marked *certified organic*. This means the produce has been cultivated according to strict uniform standards that are verified by independent state or private organizations. Certification includes inspection of farms and processing facilities, detailed record keeping, and pesticide testing of soil and water to ensure that growers and handlers are meeting government standards.

4. Support your local farms and farmers who sell their produce at farmers markets, local markets, and home deliveries.

Many of the smaller farms can't promote their wares as "organic," but if you talk with them, you'll learn that they don't use pesticides or chemical fertilizers; they just can't afford to get certified as organic. Buying your produce from a local source is also the best way to insure freshness. The fresher the vegetables and fruit, the more biophotons you'll be receiving.

5. Completely avoid irradiated foods.

Nonorganic vegetables, meats, and other products have been irradiated for years. Irradiation (exposure to radiation in very high levels) kills insects and other bugs that may have crawled into foods before being shipped to the grocery store. Irradiation has been shown to produce chromosome damage and cause nutrient destruction.[8] Food growers and manufacturers must put the irradiation symbol (radura, which is a green flower within a circle) on the label that the food is irradiated, so avoidance of irradiated foods is possible if one shops carefully.

6. Say no to genetically modified (GM) plant varieties that have been modified for herbicide tolerance and pest tolerance.[9]

When trying to avoid the top GM crops, you'll need to watch out for maltodextrin, soy lecithin, soy oil, textured vegetable protein (soy), canola oil, corn products, and high-fructose corn syrup. Other GM crops to avoid include some varieties of zucchini, crookneck squash, papayas from Hawaii, aspartame (NutraSweet), milk containing rbGH, and rennet (containing genetically modified enzymes) used to make hard cheeses.

We must become informed consumers and careful shoppers. We can look at the labels of packaged products to see if they contain corn flour or cornmeal, soy flour, cornstarch, textured vegetable protein (TVP), corn syrup, or modified food starch. Check labels of soy sauce, tofu, soy beverages, soy protein isolate, soymilk, soy ice cream, soy cheese, margarine, and soy lecithin, among dozens of other products. If it doesn't say organic or non-GMO, don't buy it;

the chances are strong that they are GMO. To shop smart, see the Non-GMO Shopping Guide, created by the Institute for Responsible Technology, at www.nongmoshoppingguide.com.

7. Wise up about red meat.

Not all red meat is created equal. In addition to being higher in omega-3 fats and CLA, meat from grass-fed animals is also higher in vitamin E. In fact, studies show the meat from pastured cattle is four times higher in vitamin E than meat from feedlot cattle and, interestingly, almost twice as high as the meat from feedlot cattle given vitamin E supplements. That's beneficial, in that vitamin E is linked with a lower risk of heart disease and cancer.[10] Grass-fed beef is also lower in total fat and particularly the saturated fats linked to heart disease. It's also higher in beta-carotene, the B vitamins thiamine and riboflavin, and the minerals calcium, magnesium, and potassium.

8. Know the difference between pastured poultry versus free-range or commercial fowl.

Pasture-raised poultry are far healthier than commercial-raised fowl. Pastured poultry are chickens, turkey, ducks, and geese that are raised in bottomless cages or pens outside or on grass where they can peck and scratch at the ground and hunt for bugs and seeds along with their grain. Sometimes they are mistakenly called free-range chickens, but free-range birds are still kept in confinement; they are just allowed to move about inside their buildings, which are often very crowded so "roaming" is not really possible.

When you choose pasture-raised chicken, you avoid hormones,

antibiotics, and drugs, which may cause immunological effects and cancer risks for consumers.[11] Commercial poultry are also often fed trace amounts of arsenic in their feed to stimulate their appetites so they'll fatten quickly for market. Traces of arsenic can be found in the meat we buy.[12]

9. Look for eggs from chickens that are raised cage-free on pasture, without hormones, and fed an organic diet that includes green grass.

Eggs from pastured hens contain all eight essential amino acids and are a rich source of essential fatty acids. They also contain considerably more lecithin (a fat emulsifier) than cholesterol. Additionally, eggs from hens bred outdoors have four to six times more vitamin D than eggs from hens bred in confinement.[13] Pastured hens are exposed to direct sunlight, which is converted to vitamin D and passed on to the eggs. And the eggs are rich in sulfur and glutathione as well.

For organic pastured eggs, look to co-ops and natural food markets; also seek out local producers, farmers, and homesteaders who pasture their poultry in movable pens or let them roam free.

10. Buy only wild-caught fish—meaning caught with a boat and hook or net.

The other option is ranched or farm-raised fish, which you should avoid. Farm-raised fish are housed within small pens that are set up in the ocean or in small ponds. The fish are often kept in overcrowded conditions that increase their risk of infection and disease. Farm-raised fish do not have the essential fatty acids that wild-caught fish offer and that are so important for our health. When it comes to animal fat, wild-caught fish are a good source of the healthy omega-3 fatty acids, especially coldwater fish such as salmon, mackerel, and trout. Also, the smaller the fish, the less mercury and other heavy metals that will be stored in the flesh and fat.

Choosing organic living foods, which means raw or dehydrated and whole foods, feeds the body superior nutrition and does not stress the body with toxins from preservatives, pesticides, and fillers. The nutrients they provide support the immune system, adrenal glands, and nervous system. As a result, we are able to better cope with stress. Studies show we will be calmer, happier, and have more energy to face daily demands. Also, avoiding foods you are sensitive to such as wheat, dairy, soy, sweets, and corn will remove a lot of stress from the body. Purchase high-quality whole foods, and you will be investing in your health—one of the best investments you could make.

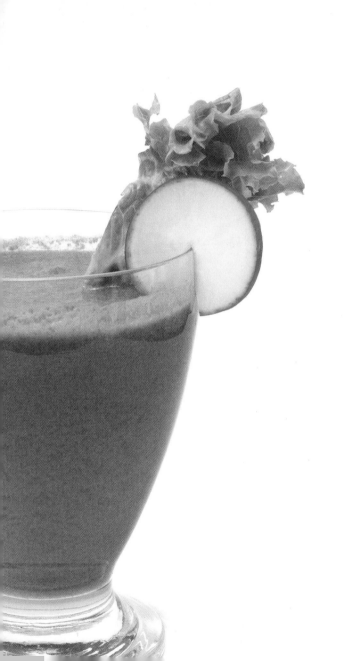

Chapter 5

BEVERAGES, FATS, and SWEETENERS—CHOOSING HEALTHY ACCESSORIES for YOUR LIVING FOODS DIET

W HAT WE DRINK is as important as what we eat. Sodas, alcohol, coffee, sports drinks, and even vitamin water can add to stress in the body due to sweeteners, artificial sweeteners, and chemicals. Conversely, organic, cold-pressed vegetable juices can support and sustain the body and promote healing and restoration. Be aware that sweeteners can negatively impact the adrenal glands. Therefore, it's wise to make healthy choices in all that we consume.

Vegetable Juice, Tea, and Other Beverages

Freshly made raw, vegetable juices are alkaline producing. Avoid processed fruit juices; they become more acid producing when processed and especially when sweetened. Fresh vegetable juices are an integral part of your living foods lifestyle regimen because they promote health in a variety of ways. The concentration of vitamins, minerals, phytonutrients, biophotons, and enzymes gives the body extra stamina and boosts the immune system.

You can juice them the night before and take the juice to work in a stainless steel water bottle or thermos. You can store juice in a covered container in the refrigerator up to twenty-four hours, forty-eight if it is cold pressed. It won't lose all its nutrients as some say, although the longer juice sits, the more nutrients it loses. You can also freeze juice. Often busy moms only have time to prepare juice on the weekend and freeze for later.

One cup of green tea is a great addition to your daily healthy lifestyle. Rich in antioxidants and the phytonutrients catechins and other polyphenols that protect against inflammation, cancer, and other ailments, green tea is also thermogenic. Thermogenesis is the production of heat, meaning that it revs up your metabolism. Most of the thermogenic action in green tea is due to epigallocatechin gallate (EGCG), which is a potent polyphenol.

A cup of green tea has about one-third of the caffeine found in a cup of coffee. However, you need to avoid green tea if you are sensitive to caffeine, have low adrenal function, or are hypoglycemic.

White tea has less caffeine than green tea and may be better tolerated. Herbal teas are also a great choice and are fine for those with low adrenal function and who are hypoglycemic. When choosing green, white, and herbal tea, look for organically grown. Also unbleached tea bags are a better choice over bleached.

For sparkling water, choose mineral water that is naturally carbonated such as S. Pellegrino and Apollinaris over commercially gassed varieties. If you suffer from IBS (irritable bowel syndrome), Crohn's disease, celiac, or diverticulitis, it is advisable to completely eliminate carbonated drinks along with all gluten from your diet in order to allow the GI lining of your intestinal tract to heal.

Be sure to drink plenty of water. It's recommended that you drink at least eight 8-ounce glasses of purified water per day to maintain good health. A good water purifier is a great investment. Be aware of plastic toxins that are leached into the water from plastic bottles. Take water with you in stainless steel water bottles.

Completely avoid soft drinks; they are like drinking liquid candy with chemicals so caustic they can rust nails. They're loaded with sugar or artificial sweeteners, which are even worse. Studies have connected them with weight gain and numerous health problems. They're also very acidic. Also, watch out for sweetened teas, energy drinks, sports drinks, and vitamin-infused water (usually loaded with sweeteners). And always avoid diet sodas due to their detrimental health effects. NutraSweet (aspartame) has been linked with brain tumors.[1] Also studies show artificial sweeteners actually cause people to gain weight.[2]

Shopping Guide for Healthy Fats and Oils

For decades we've have had a love-hate relationship with this food that makes so many dishes taste great. Fat gives us that feeling of satisfaction we all long for—satiety, which is the sense that we've had enough to eat. But that's not all. Fats play an important role in our body's health. Some fats can even help us lose weight. We also need fats to absorb fat-soluble vitamins such as A, D, E, and K.

When people eat foods prepared with processed vegetable oils— margarine, french fries, fried food, nonfat dried milk, powdered or liquid coffee creamer, many salad dressings, crackers, cookies, chips, and a plethora of processed and convenience foods—they eat a high quantity of oxidized (rancid) oil. This sets the body up for heart disease and numerous other health problems.

ACAI AND OTHER BERRIES HELP DEFEND AGAINST LIFE'S STRESSORS

Acai berries are inch-long reddish-purple fruit. They come from the acai palm tree, which is native to Central and South America. Research has examined their antioxidant activity 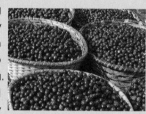 because antioxidants can help prevent diseases caused by oxidative stress, such as heart disease and cancer. Acai berries contain substances known as anthocyanins and flavonoids. Anthocyanins cause the red, purple, and blue shades in many fruits and vegetables. The foods richest in anthocyanins such as blueberries, red grapes, and acai range from deep purple to black. Some studies show that acai has even more antioxidant content than cranberries, raspberries, blackberries, strawberries, and blueberries.[3]

Anthocyanins and flavonoids are potent antioxidants that help defend us against life's stressors. They also have a role in cell protection by quenching free radicals—harmful products that damage cells. When we include plenty of antioxidant-rich fruits and vegetables in our diets, we slow down the aging process and prevent disease by neutralizing free radicals.

To help you choose the very best oils and fats, use the following shopping guide for the healthiest fats and oils, along with the ones to avoid. I've also included the smoke point of the oils recommended, which is the point at which fat breaks down, starts to smoke, and gives off an odor, signaling the oxidation of these oils.

Coconut oil. Choose only organic virgin coconut oil, which means it has been made by a traditional method that does not involve high heat or harmful chemicals. It won't oxidize (turn rancid) as easily because it doesn't have the double bonds that make polyunsaturated oils most vulnerable to oxidation. It has a longer shelf life (about two years) than most oils and does not need to be refrigerated. It has been a staple cooking oil for thousands of years in tropical climates. It is white when solid, creamy colored when liquid. You will pay more for this oil, but it's well worth it.

Research has shown that coconut oil can help you lose weight—the body likes to burn its medium-chain fatty acids rather than store them as it does long-chain fatty acids that dominate most other oils.[4] It has a "thermogenic effect," meaning it raises body temperature, thus boosting energy and metabolic rate and promoting weight loss. It has also been shown in a university study to kill yeasts, even Candida albicans.[5]

Coconut oil is great for medium-heat cooking (smoke point of 350 degrees). It has no cholesterol, which some have claimed. And it tastes great on popcorn as well as everything else.

Olive oil is an outstanding monounsaturated fat. A tablespoon of extra-virgin olive oil contains 11 grams of monounsaturated fat, 2 grams of saturated fat, and 1 gram of polyunsaturated fat. An ancient oil dating back to biblical times, it was used for cooking and healing. It is more shelf stable than polyunsaturated oils. The most flavorful, healthful, and eco-friendly varieties are extra-virgin, organic oils that are cold-pressed or expeller-pressed. These are produced without chemical solvents like hexane and high heat. High-quality olive oil stands out also as an antioxidant that is a free-radical fighter.

Olive oil is great for salad dressings, cold foods, and low-heat cooking such as light sautéing. Extra-virgin olive oil has a smoke point of 305–320 degrees. Completely avoid the less expensive, chemically derived version called olive pomace oil—the last dregs of the olive oil pressing process, extracted by petroleum solvents such as hexane.

Almond oil is monounsaturated oil that is extracted from the almond and has a distinctively nutty flavor. It is typically used as an ingredient in salad dressings, sauces, mayonnaise, baked goods, and desserts. Unlike almond extract, almond oil is not concentrated enough to provide a strong almond taste. It is suited for high-heat cooking and baking with a smoke point of 420 degrees. Many toxic pesticides and herbicides are used on almond trees; therefore, choose only organic cold-pressed or expeller-pressed almond oil.

Avocado oil is extracted from the avocado by pressing the flesh, not the seed. It is often compared to olive oil because the oils are similar in composition, but avocado oil has a much higher smoke point of 520 degrees and is good for high-heat cooking and baking. High-quality avocado oil has a distinct green color due to its chlorophyll content. It also has a characteristic avocado flavor, depending on how the oil has been processed and handled and the quality of the avocados used. Avocado oil is fairly shelf stable and does not oxidize easily. Choose cold-pressed or expeller-pressed avocado oil. Avoid chemically processed oil altogether. It is not necessary to purchase organic avocado oil since avocado is on the clean fifteen list (see ewg.org).

Rice bran oil is extracted from the germ and inner husk of rice. It is dominantly monounsaturated. A tablespoon contains 7 grams of monounsaturated fat, 3 grams of saturated fat, and 5 grams of polyunsaturated fat. It contains healthful phytochemicals such as beta-sitosterol, which can reduce the absorption of cholesterol, and alpha-linoleic acid, which can increase essential fatty acid concentration.

Rice bran oil has a mild taste with a smoke point of 490 degrees, making it perfect for stir-frying. It is said to be the secret of good tempura. Rice bran oil also contains components of vitamin E that may benefit health and prevent rancidity. Look for organic, cold-pressed or expeller-pressed oil.

Peanut oil (unrefined) has a smoke point of 320 degrees, which makes it good for only low-heat cooking. Refined peanut oil has a much higher smoke point but is not recommended because of being refined. Peanut oil contains 48 percent monounsaturated fat, 18 percent saturated fat, and 34 percent polyunsaturated fat. Like olive oil, peanut oil is relatively stable and, therefore, appropriate for stir-fry. But the high percentage of omega-6 fatty acids it contains presents a potential problem since the American diet contains far too much omega-6 already and not enough omega-3 fats. Also peanuts are a goitrogen, meaning they block iodine absorption, which can promote low thyroid function.

Limit your use of peanut oil, and choose only organic, cold-pressed, or expeller-pressed, or better yet, avoid it altogether since peanuts are grown underground and known to absorb toxins from the soil.

Sesame oil contains 42 percent monounsaturated fat, 15 percent saturated fat, and 43 percent polyunsaturated fat. It has been used for thousands of years in Asian culture. Sesame oil is similar in composition to peanut oil. The high percentage of omega-6 fats indicates that it should be used only occasionally in small quantities. Hexane is typically used to extract oil from the seeds, so choose only cold-pressed or expeller-pressed oil, and always refrigerate it. Organic is better, but pesticide residues are minor in nonorganic sesame seeds and oils.

Macadamia nut oil is expressed from the meat of the macadamia. Native to Australia, the oil contains approximately 60 percent monounsaturated fat, about 20 percent saturated fat, and 20 percent polyunsaturated fat. Some varieties contain roughly equal omega-6s and omega-3s. It is very shelf stable due to its low polyunsaturated fat content. It has a smoke point of 410 degrees, making it suitable for higher-heat cooking and baking. Few pesticides are used on these nuts, so organic oil is not necessary. But choose only cold-pressed or expeller-pressed oil because the highest concentration of hexane residue was found in macadamia nut oil in a study that tested 41 samples of vegetable, fruit, and nut oils.[6]

Butter. Purchase organic butter made from the milk of grass-fed cows. It has more cancer-fighting conjugated linoleic acid (CLA), vitamin E, beta-carotene, and omega-3 fatty acids than butter from cows raised on factory farms or that have limited access to pasture. It is a rich source of vitamins A, E, K, and D. It also has appreciable amounts of butyric acid, which is used by the colon as an energy source, and lauric acid, a medium-chain fatty acid that is a potent antimicrobial and antifungal substance. The naturally golden color of grass-fed butter is a good indication of its superior nutritional value.[7]

Butter is suited for medium-heat cooking with a smoke point of 350 degrees. Ghee, which is clarified butter, has a smoke point between 375 and 485 degrees and is good for medium- to high-heat cooking.

Avoid These Foods Completely

Polyunsaturated oils. In their natural state, as found in nuts, vegetables, and seeds, polyunsaturated fats are healthy. But when they are processed into oil, they oxidize easily and do more harm than good. They promote inflammation that leads to weight gain, depression, and immune system dysfunction. Completely avoid corn, soy, sunflower, and safflower oils.

Canola oil is a monounsaturated fat, as is olive oil, which means it contains only one double bond, so technically it could be used for salad dressings, cold food preparation, and low-temperature cooking. But there's a major reason not to use it: most canola oil comes from GM crops. Also, researchers at the University of

Florida at Gainesville found trans fat levels as high as 4.6 percent in processed canola oil.[8]

Trans fats are created in the process of hydrogenating oils and should be avoided completely. The consumption of trans fats increases the risk of coronary heart disease. Commercially baked goods such as crackers, cookies, cakes, muffins, and many fried foods, such as doughnuts and french fries, may contain trans fats. Mainstream shortenings and some margarine can be high in trans fat.

Margarine and butter replacement spreads. Margarine is made from different types of oils that often are hydrogenated—a process used to solidify them, making the margarine solid and spreadable. The *New York Times* says, "A new report by Harvard researchers says a fat [trans fat] in margarine and other processed foods could be responsible for 30,000 of the nation's annual deaths from heart disease."[9] When it comes to natural spreads that are substitutes for butter, read labels; know what oils are used. An olive oil or coconut oil spread would be fine, unless it is hydrogenated, but anything made with polyunsaturated oils should be avoided, and/or canola oil (unless it specifically says non-GMO/no trans fats) should be avoided.

Salt. Choose only Celtic sea salt, Himalayan pink, or gray salt. Whole sea salt has a mineral profile that is similar to our blood. Regular table salt is highly refined sodium chloride that usually contains additives to make it pour easily. When salt is processed, minerals are removed. Then, anti-caking chemicals such as potassium oxide or aluminum calcium silicate, iodine, and dextrose (sugar) are added to make table salt.

Sugar—all types. Many health professionals attribute it to the increase in obesity, metabolic syndrome, diabetes, certain cancers, and heart disease. All of these sugar sources need to be avoided: high-fructose corn syrup, sucrose (white sugar—another big GMO product), brown sugar (white sugar with molasses added), dextrose (produced synthetically from starch), agave syrup, dextrin (a complex sugar molecule left over from enzyme action on starch), sugar alcohols such as sorbitol and manitol, xylitol (choose only organic from birch trees—much of the xylitol on the market is made from by-products of the wood pulp industry or from cane pulp, seed hulls, or cornhusk), evaporated cane juice, cane sugar, sucanat, and molasses. The more you avoid sugar, the less you will crave it. And you'll lose weight!

Artificial sweeteners. Completely avoid all artificial sweeteners (NutraSweet, Splenda, Sweet 'n Low, Equal), which can cause a host of health problems. And if you think they're helping you lose weight, take a look at the research. People on sugar substitutes actually gain more weight than those using sugar.[10] And using sugar is a very bad choice for your weight as well as your health, but the artificial sweeteners are even worse.

Long-term use can create a ticking time bomb for a large array of neurological illnesses, including (but not limited to) brain cancer, Lou Gehrig's disease, Graves' disease, chronic fatigue syndrome, multiple sclerosis (MS), and epilepsy.[11]

Sweeteners to use sparingly include raw unfiltered local honey, brown rice syrup, and pure maple syrup. I recommend stevia as the best sweetener to use.

For years I have said, "Change your diet and you can change your life!" My health didn't take a real turn for the best until I gave up sweeteners and started juicing. The healthiest beverage on earth, apart from pure water, is vegetable juice. When I'm on vacation, I truly notice a difference in not having it every day. I can't wait to get back to my healthy juicing routine. Choosing healthy fats is also an excellent choice that can make a big difference in your health. We've come through the decades of low-fat and no-fat teaching. In place of fat, people were encouraged to add sweeteners or fruit. All this sugar taxed the body, caused many cravings, and set us up for diseases such as diabetes or certain cancers. Now that you know the truth, you can make wise choices and heal your entire body, including your adrenal glands.

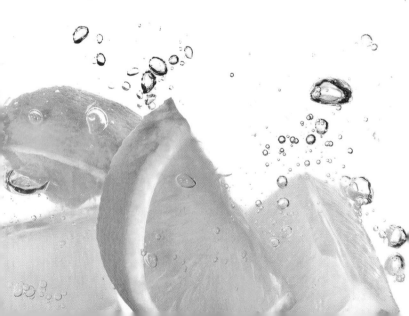

Chapter 6

THE LIVING FOODS MEAL PLAN to SUPPORT YOUR ADRENAL GLANDS

THERE ARE TWO menu plans in this section—the all-raw menu plan and a menu plan with some cooked vegan foods and some animal products. You can adapt either menu plan to fit your needs. Whichever menu plan you choose, make sure you include some protein, especially in the morning.

You will drink two glasses of vegetable juice each day. Make fresh juice whenever you can. If you can't make fresh juice, you can buy it at a juice bar. You may have more than two glasses of vegetable juice a day, but not less. The time of day you drink the juice is up to you. Many people like to start their day with fresh juice to energize their minds and bodies, while others take juice to work in a glass or stainless steel water bottle or thermos and drink it midmorning as a pick-me-up.

The other glass of juice should be consumed either midafternoon or before dinner. A juice of choice is listed for breakfast with a juice of choice as optional midmorning. The same goes for the afternoon. This does not mean you need to drink two glasses of juice in the morning and two glasses in the afternoon, unless you desire; the options are there so you can choose the time that fits best. And recipes are listed just to give you an idea of the recipes available to you. This in no way means that you have to drink that recipe at that time. Choose the recipes you like and fit them into your menu plan.

The following menu plan is simply a guideline to help you see how you can plan your days. You can use the recipes and ideas in this chapter or choose your own that fit the adrenal restoration guidelines for healthy eating. Remember, that means keep the refined and starchy carbohydrates along with gluten out of your diet and completely avoid refined and processed foods.

When you are tired, the tendency is to reach for instant energy foods such as cookies, ice cream, cake, doughnuts, bread, pasta, coffee, soda, or an energy drink. However, the "energy" you get from these choices is false; they cause a dip in energy a little later after consumption that makes you feel worse in the end.

Be aware that people with adrenal fatigue often crave salt. In people with adrenal insufficiency, salt cravings are mostly due to low levels of aldosterone (steroid hormone). Like cortisol, aldosterone is produced by the adrenal cortex. Aldosterone is part of a complex system that regulates blood pressure, partly by helping the body to hang on to salt and water. Levels of aldosterone go up and down in a daily pattern similar to cortisol. It is significantly influenced by stress. Usually when cortisol goes up, aldosterone goes down, which lowers blood pressure. If cortisol levels stay high, or your adrenal glands run down, chronically low aldosterone can disturb both electrolyte balance and cell hydration. Therefore, increasing your salt intake is one way to help restore such imbalances. Make sure you choose only good quality salt such as Celtic sea salt.

Must-Have Kitchen Equipment to Properly Prepare Your Living Foods

First we are going to look at what tools you will need in your live foods kitchen and how to properly prepare your foods to maintain the highest quality of nutrients for your body. There are several kitchen equipment items that will make your food preparation much easier. A juicer and blender are a must to own, and the other items will help you make great food you can enjoy so that you will be more inclined to stick with your living foods lifestyle.

- *Juicer.* A good juicer that is easy to use and clean is the main tool in your health and healing diet. If you don't have a juicer or are unhappy with the one you have, and you're wondering which juicer is right for you, you can check out juicers on my website at www.juiceladycherie.com.

- *Blender.* A blender is needed to make the great raw soups and savory smoothie recipes. But you don't have to spend a lot of money to get a good blender. Most blenders work just fine. The top of the line is the Vita Mix, which does a tremendous job.

- *Dehydrator.* Though a dehydrator is not necessary to make a healthy diet work, it's a great appliance that enables you to make delicious low-calorie, low-glycemic snacks. For more information on dehydrators, visit www.juiceladycherie.com.

- *Spiral slicer or spirooli slicer.* The spiral slicer, originally from Japan, is used to make raw spaghetti dishes, thin slices for dehydrated veggies, and curls for decorative salads and dishes. (The raw spaghetti is more like linguini width with the spiral slicer.) The spirooli is a three-in-one turning slicer for vegetables; it slices, shreds, and chips veggies on a rotating arm. It makes a thicker noodle strand than the spiral slicer—more like spaghetti width. You can turn almost any vegetable into spaghetti-type strands, slices, or julienne strips, such as onion, zucchini, carrot, cucumber, turnip, potato, sweet potato, daikon radish, and butternut squash.

- *Mandolin food slicer* makes crinkle cuts, thin uniform slices, and julienne strips in a variety of thicknesses. The blade ensures even soft foods such as tomatoes slice perfectly. This tool is very helpful to make thin slices for dehydrated foods and raw dishes.

The Best Way to Cook Your Food

Unless you go all-raw vegan, as some people have, you'll want to cook or warm up leftovers in the healthiest way possible. How you do that is extremely important to your health. That's why I'm recommending that you only use your stovetop, oven, toaster oven, countertop grill, or convection oven. I think when you finish reading the data I've collected, you'll want to toss out your microwave for good reasons.

It has been found that radiation exposure can weaken the immune system and cause health-related problems such as cancer and degenerative diseases. It may also cause ailments such as "persistent cough, headaches, sleep disturbances, and gastrointestinal dysfunction," notes Dr. J. D. Decuypere. She has observed that respiratory illnesses such as asthma, bronchitis, chronic cough, and allergies have been increasing since the late 1970s, which prompted her to do her own investigation on radiation in our food.[1]

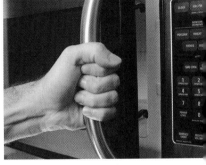

Though there are numerous ways that we are exposed to radiation, there are two ways that it enters our food—microwave ovens and irradiation of food. Radiating food in a microwave oven is convenient, and many people use their microwaves daily. But studies have shown that it may negatively impact the nutrition of the food, and it may be harmful to the people who eat it.

The British medical journal *The Lancet* (December 9, 1989) reported that when microwaving baby bottles, "one of the amino acids, L-proline, was converted to its d-isomer, which is known to be neurotoxic and nephrotoxic. It's bad enough that many babies are not nursed. Now they are given fake milk (baby formula) made even more toxic by microwaving."[2]

The radiation process of a microwave oven can alter a food's molecular structure and create new chemicals called unique radiolytic products (URPs). If that sounds harmless to you, then you need to know that URPs include benzene, formaldehyde, and a host of mutagens and carcinogens—a fact that should alert you to the potential hazards of eating microwaved foods.[3]

A study performed by Dr. Hans Hertel of Switzerland found that food prepared in microwave ovens had molecular alteration, but he found too that it also altered the blood chemistry of people eating it. Volunteers had:

- Altered hemoglobin and cholesterol values, especially HDL and LDL values and ratio

- Lymphocytes (white blood cells) that demonstrated a more distinct short-term decrease following consumption of microwaved food than after eating anything else. Dr. Hertel said these changes point toward degeneration of health. The natural repair mechanisms of cells become disturbed, which forces cells to respond to a "state-of-emergency" energy supply, exchanging aerobic (oxygen-based) for anaerobic (no oxygen) respiration. This constitutes a cancer-type effect on the blood—cancer cells are anaerobic.[4]

Here are some of the results of various studies on microwaving foods:

- Creation of d-Nitrosodiethanolamines—a cancer-causing agent

- Creation of cancer-causing agents within protein compounds in milk and cereal grains

- Alteration in the breakdown of glucoside and galactoside elements within frozen fruits when thawed in a microwave oven

- Altered catabolic behavior of plant alkaloids when raw, cooked, or frozen vegetables were microwave heated for even a short time

- Cancer-causing free radicals formed within certain trace-mineral molecular formations in plants, especially in raw root vegetables

- A higher percentage of cancerous cells in the blood

- Malfunctions occurring in the lymphatic system, causing degeneration of the immune system's capacity to protect itself against cancerous growth

- Altered food substances leading to disorders in the digestive system

- A statistically higher incidence of stomach and intestinal cancers, plus a general degeneration of peripheral cellular tissues with a gradual breakdown of digestive and excretory system function

- Significant decrease in the nutritional value of all foods studied

- A decrease in the availability of B-complex vitamins, vitamin C, vitamin E, essential minerals, and lipotropic nutrients

- Destruction of the nutritional value of protein in meat

- Lowering of the metabolic activity of alkaloids, glucosides, galactosides, and nitrilosides (basic plant substances in fruits and vegetables)

- Marked acceleration of structural disintegration in all foods[5]

Microwaving food in plastic containers poses an additional risk of the food absorbing dangerous chemicals released from the plastic when it is heated. While the dangers of using microwave ovens are still embroiled in battle and controversy, it is highly recommended that you not use a microwave at all—even for heating water. Recently a friend sent an e-mail to me about a woman who conducted a home experiment with two similar plants. She watered one with cooled microwaved water and the other with tap water. The microwave-watered plant died rather quickly.

Now that you know how to maintain the highest level of nutrients in your foods and have the right tools for the job, let me give an example of what one day of meals should look like as you use nature's bounty to rebuild your stressed adrenals and bring balance back to your body.

Sample diet plan (Day 1)

Upon rising

Start your day with ⅛ to ½ teaspoon of Celtic sea salt or kelp powder dissolved in a glass of water, juice, or herbal tea. Drink another glass at your lowest energy point during the day. When the adrenal glands are fatigued, they do not produce enough aldosterone. Aldosterone regulates the amount of sodium and potassium in the body. When aldosterone becomes deficient, not enough salt is retained in the body. Have you been craving salt? This is probably the reason.

Avoid caffeine

Coffee, black tea, and possibly even green tea for a while (although it has ⅓ the caffeine of coffee) should be avoided. Even white tea, which has the least caffeine of all, may be too much for your weak adrenals. Pushing your adrenals with caffeine is like whipping a tired horse that needs to rest.

Breakfast

Try the Adrenal Booster Cocktail followed by a Healthy Green Smoothie. Eat some protein following your juice or smoothie, such as a boiled egg.

Midmorning or midafternoon

Have a fresh glass of vegetable juice midmorning and/or mid- to late afternoon. Dark green juices are particularly beneficial.

Lunch and dinner

Raw foods are helpful in healing the body because of their superior nutrients and biophotons. You can choose raw food recipes, some cooked food recipes, and some animal products that are organic, grass fed, and free range, if you are not vegan. Eat plenty of high-fiber vegetables. There is a need for high-quality protein as well. You may need some animal protein for a while unless you go mostly raw and really focus on getting enough high-quality protein from seeds, nuts, sprouts, and dark leafy greens. You may also need to supplement with free-form amino acids. The amino acid program has made a significant difference for many people I've worked with. Also, keep your blood sugar balanced. Eat smaller meals and a couple of very nutritious snacks during the day.

Nutrients and juices (daily recommendations)

Vitamin C
2,000–5,000 mg/day with bioflavonoids (you may actually need more vitamin C for a while)
Foods to juice: hot peppers, kale, parsley, collard, turnip greens, broccoli, mustard greens, watercress, lemons with white part, and spinach

Vitamin E
800 IU/day with mixed tocopherols
Foods to juice: spinach, asparagus, and carrots

Niacin
125–150 mg/day, as niacinamide

Pyridoxine (vitamin B_6)
150 mg/day
Foods to juice: spinach, kale, and avocado, which can't be juiced but is good in green smoothies

Pantothenic acid (vitamin B_5)
1,200–1,500 mg/day
Foods to juice: broccoli and kale

Vitamin B-100 Complex
I suggest B Complex 12 by Thorne; take as directed.

Magnesium citrate
400–1,200 mg/day
Foods to juice: beet greens, spinach, parsley, dandelion greens, garlic, beets, carrots, celery, and avocado (green smoothies)

Trace minerals
Multi-minerals; they have a calming effect
I suggest Citramins (multi-minerals) by Thorne; take as directed.
Foods to juice: Dark leafy greens are especially rich in minerals.

Herbs

Rhodiola rosea
Enhances memory and concentration; has been shown to reduce stress-induced fatigue and improve mental performance

Holy basil leaf
Helps to normalize cortisol in times of stress

Wild oats milky seed
Supports the nervous system

Schisandra berry
Helps with energy, endurance, and resistance to stress

Ashwagandha
Has been shown to have a sedating effect on the body and helps to rebuild the digestive and nervous system

Siberian ginseng

Has been used traditionally to stimulate and nourish the adrenal glands and increases mental alertness

Cordyceps

A Chinese mushroom used for supporting the adrenal gland; can also help the immune function

Licorice root (not the candy)

Provides a lift for the adrenal glands and improves resistance to stress; should be used in small amounts according to directions since it can raise blood pressure in higher quantities

MAGNESIUM: NATURE'S VALIUM

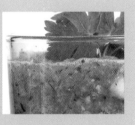

Juice your greens—they're rich in magnesium, known as nature's Valium! Magnesium is critical for more than three hundred chemical reactions in your body, and unfortunately most Americans are deficient in this mineral. In fact, it may be the single most important nutritional deficiency in the United States.

Many studies have shown that even a small amount of magnesium has a major effect on preventing heart attacks. Magnesium also has been called the "antistress mineral." It plays a vital role in fighting off stress, relaxes muscles, prevents osteoporosis, builds healthy bones, supports restful sleep, prevents restless leg syndrome, prevents constipation, boosts energy, calms the body, and relieves tension.

Magnesium also helps us lose weight. A lack of magnesium is a definite contributor to weight gain and obesity. When magnesium is low, cells don't recognize insulin and glucose accumulates in the blood—then it gets stored as fat instead of being burned for fuel. Further, magnesium helps prevent fat storage.

When magnesium levels drop too low, it can trigger hyperventilation and panic attacks, even seizures, if severe. Such symptoms can be relieved by increasing dietary magnesium. You can take magnesium supplements, but make sure you use only absorbable forms such as magnesium citrate or glycinate. The particles in magnesium supplements are too large for the body to completely absorb, which makes the magnesium in green juice far superior.

Green plants take inorganic minerals from the soil through their tiny roots and incorporate them into their cells, turning them into very absorbable organic minerals. These mineral 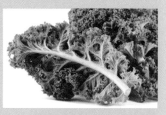 particles are much smaller and easier for the body to absorb than those found in supplements. It is estimated that more than 90 percent of a plant's minerals is delivered to the cells when you juice greens. So juice up the beautiful leaves of these magnesium-rich greens:

- Chard
- Collards
- Beet tops
- Parsley
- Spinach
- Kohlrabi leaves
- Kale
- Dandelion greens
- Lettuce (dark green)
- Mustard greens

And here's more good news—you'll increase your energy exponentially. That means you'll actually get more done rather than stressing about getting more done. You also feel more like working out, which is another great stress-busting habit.

If you take your adrenal treatment plan seriously, you can expect your adrenal fatigue to heal in:

- Six to nine months for minor adrenal fatigue
- Twelve to eighteen months for moderate adrenal fatigue
- Twenty-four to thirty-six months for severe adrenal fatigue

The most important factor is not to give up, even when you don't see immediate results. Stick with the program and keep up your healthy lifestyle choices. There is a reward of good health and energy in the end.

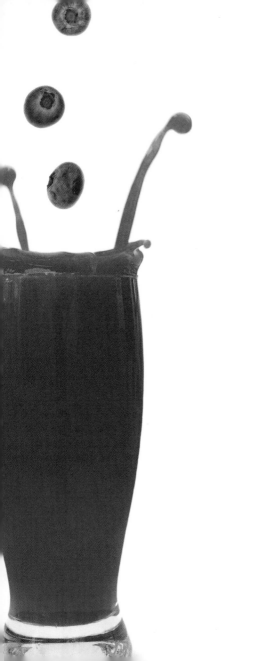

Chapter 7

BEST TIPS for MAKING FRESH JUICES and SMOOTHIES

EVERY TIME YOU pour a glass of juice, picture a big vitamin-mineral cocktail with a wealth of nutrients that promote adrenal health and vitality. The veggies are broken down into an easily absorbable form that your body can use—right away. This food doesn't have to go through a big process of breaking everything down. So it goes to work in your body to give you energy and renew you right down to your cells. It also spares your organs all the work it takes to digest food, and that equates to more energy. It detoxifies your body as well because it's rich in antioxidants, so that lightens your toxic load, and the body doesn't have to work so hard to deal with all the toxic stuff coming from the environment.

The Nutritional Components of Fresh Juice

In addition to water and easily absorbed protein and carbohydrates, juice also provides essential fatty acids, vitamins, minerals, enzymes, biophotons, and phytonutrients. And researchers are continuing to explore how the nutrients found in juice help the body heal and shed unwanted pounds. The next time you make a glass of fresh juice, this is what you'll be drinking:

Protein

When you think of protein sources, does juice ever come to mind? Probably not, but surprisingly it does offer more than you might think. We use protein to form muscles, ligaments, tendons, hair, nails, and skin. Protein is needed to create enzymes, which direct chemical reactions, and hormones, which guide bodily functions. Fruits and vegetables contain lower quantities of protein than animal foods such as muscle meats and dairy products. Therefore they are thought of as poor protein sources. But juices are concentrated forms of vegetables and fruit and so provide easily absorbed amino acids, the building blocks that make up protein. For example, 16 ounces of carrot juice (2 to 3 pounds of carrots) provide about 5 grams of protein (the equivalent of about one chicken wing or 2 ounces of tofu). Vegetable protein is not complete protein, so it does not provide all the amino acids your body needs. In addition to lots of dark leafy greens, you'll want to eat other protein sources, such as sprouts, legumes (beans, lentils, and split peas), nuts, seeds, and whole grains. If you're not vegan, you can add eggs and free-range, grass-fed muscle meats such as chicken, turkey, lamb, and beef along with wild-caught fish.

Carbohydrates

Vegetable and fruit juices contain carbohydrates. Carbs provide fuel for the body, which uses it for movement, heat production, and chemical reactions. The chemical bonds of carbohydrates lock in the energy a plant takes up from the sun, and this energy is released when the body burns plant food as fuel. There are three categories of carbs: simple (sugars), complex (starches and fiber), and fiber.

Choose more complex carbohydrates than simple carbs in your diet. There are more simple sugars in fruit juice than vegetable juice, which is why you should juice more vegetables and in most cases drink no more than 4 ounces of fruit juice a day. Both insoluble and soluble fibers are found in whole fruits and vegetables, and both types are needed for good health. Who said juice doesn't have fiber? Juice has the soluble form—pectin and gums, which are excellent for the digestive tract. Soluble fiber also helps to lower blood cholesterol levels, stabilize blood sugar, and improve good bowel bacteria.

Essential fatty acids

There is very little fat in fruit and vegetable juices, but the fats juice does contain are essential to your health. The essential fatty acids (EFAs)—linoleic and alpha-linolenic acids in particular—found in fresh juice function as components of nerve cells, cellular membranes, and hormonelike substances called prostaglandins. They are also required for energy production.

Vitamins

Fresh juice is loaded with vitamins. Vitamins take part, along with minerals and enzymes, in chemical reactions. For example, vitamin C participates in the production of collagen, one of the main types of protein found in the body. Fresh juices are excellent sources of water-soluble vitamins such as C; many of the B vitamins and some fat-soluble vitamins such as vitamin E; the carotenes, known as provitamin A (they are converted to vitamin A as needed by the body); and vitamin K. They also come packaged with cofactors, such as vitamin C with bioflavonoids. The cofactors and vitamins help each other be more effective.

Minerals

Fresh juice is loaded with minerals. There are about two dozen minerals that your body needs to function well. Minerals, along with vitamins, are components of enzymes. They make up part of bones, teeth, and blood tissue, and they help maintain normal cellular function.

The major minerals include calcium, chloride, magnesium, phosphorus, potassium, sodium, and sulfur. Trace minerals are those needed in very small amounts, which include boron, chromium, cobalt, copper, fluoride, manganese, nickel, selenium, vanadium, and zinc.

Minerals occur in inorganic forms in the soil, and plants incorporate them into their tissues. As a part of this process, the minerals are combined with organic molecules into easily absorbable forms, which make plant food an excellent dietary source of minerals. Juicing is believed to provide even better mineral absorption than whole vegetables because the process of juicing liberates minerals into a highly absorbable, easily digestible form.

Enzymes

Fresh juices are chock-full of enzymes—those "living" molecules that work with vitamins and minerals to speed up reactions necessary for vital functions in the body. Without enzymes we would not have life in our cells. Enzymes are prevalent in raw foods, but heat such as cooking and pasteurization destroys them. All juices that are bottled, even if kept in store refrigerators, have to be pasteurized. Heat temperatures for pasteurization are required to be far above the limit of what would preserve the enzymes and vitamins.

When you eat and drink enzyme-rich foods, these little proteins help break down food in the digestive tract, thereby sparing the pancreas, small intestine, and stomach—the body's enzyme producers—from overwork. This sparing action is known as the "law of adaptive secretion of digestive enzymes." According to this law, when a portion of the food you eat is digested by enzymes present in the food, the body will secrete less of its own enzymes. This allows the body's energy to be shifted from digestion to other functions such as repair and rejuvenation. Fresh juices require very little energy expenditure to digest, and that is one reason people who start consistently drinking fresh juice often report that they feel better and more energized right away.

Phytochemicals

Plants contain substances that protect them from disease, injury, and pollution. These substances are known as phytochemicals. *Phyto* means "plant," and *chemical* in this context means "nutrient." There are tens of thousands of phytochemicals in the foods we eat. For example, the average tomato may contain up to ten thousand different types of phytochemicals, the most famous being lycopene.

Phytochemicals give plants their color, odor, and flavor. Unlike vitamins and enzymes, they are heat stable and can withstand cooking. Researchers have found that people who eat the most fruits and vegetables, which are the best sources of phytochemicals, have the lowest incidence of cancer and other diseases. Drinking freshly made vegetable juices gives you these vital substances in a concentrated form.

Biophotons

There's one more substance, more difficult to measure than the others, that's present in raw foods. It is being studied scientifically in tubes and is named biophotons. It's light energy that the plants absorb from the sun, and it is found in the living cells of raw foods such as fruits and vegetables. Photons have been shown to emit coherent light energy when uniquely photographed (using Kirlian photography). This light energy is believed to have many benefits when consumed; one in particular is thought to aid cellular communication. Biophotons feed the mitochondria of the cells, which produce ATP—our body's energy fuel. Biophotons are also believed to contribute to our energy, vitality, and a feeling of vibrancy and well-being.

Frequently Asked Questions

Now that you know why juice is so effective for good health, you may have some questions about juicing. Below I will address some of the questions I am most commonly asked about juicing.

Why juice? Why not just eat the fruits and vegetables?

Though I always tell people to eat their vegetables and fruit, there are at least three reasons juice is important and should also be included in the diet. First, we can juice far more produce than we would probably eat in a day. It takes a long time to chew raw veggies. Chewing is a very good thing. I highly encourage it. However, we have only so much time for chewing raw foods. One day I timed how long it would take for me to eat five medium-size carrots. (That's what I often juice along with cucumber, lemon, ginger root, beet, kale, and celery.) It was about fifty minutes of chewing. Not only do I not have that kind of time every day, but also my jaw was so tired afterward that I could hardly move it.

Secondly, we can juice parts of the plant we would not normally eat, such as stems, leaves, and seeds. I juice things I know I would rarely or never eat, such as beet stems and leaves, celery leaves, the white pithy part of the lemon with the seeds, asparagus stems, broccoli stems, the base of cauliflower, kohlrabi leaves, radish leaves, and ribs of kale.

Thirdly, juice is broken down, so it spares digestion. It is estimated that juice is at work in the system in about twenty to thirty minutes after it is consumed. When we have ailments, juice is therapy for this very reason. When the body has to work hard to break down veggies, for example, it can spend a lot of energy on the digestive process.

Juicing does the work for you. So when you drink a glass of fresh juice, all those life-giving nutrients can go to work right away to heal and repair your body, giving it energy for its work of rejuvenation.

JUICING RECOMMENDATIONS FOR DIABETICS AND PREDIABETICS

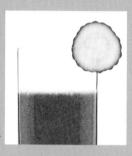

I've often heard people say they can't juice because they have diabetes. You can juice vegetables if you have sugar metabolism problems, but you should choose low-sugar veggies and only low-sugar fruits such as lemons, limes, and cranberries. Carrots and beets would be too high in sugar. You could add one or two carrots to a juice recipe or a very small beet or part of a beet, but they should be diluted with cucumber juice and dark leafy greens. You may use cranberries, lemons, and limes, but other fruits are higher in sugar and should be avoided. Berries are low in sugar, especially blueberries, and can be added to juice recipes.

Green apples are lower in sugar than yellow or red apples. But I don't recommend that you use even green apples unless you have your blood sugar under control. Keep your juices very low in sugar.

I've worked with people who have reversed their diabetes by juicing low-sugar vegetables and eating many more living foods, along with a low-glycemic, high-fiber diet.

Sprinkle cinnamon in your juice

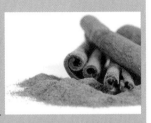

Researchers have suggested that people with diabetes may see improvements by adding ¼ to 1 teaspoon of cinnamon to their food. A twelve-week London study involved fifty-eight type 2 diabetics. After twelve weeks on 2 grams (about ½ teaspoon) of cinnamon per day, study subjects had significantly lowered blood sugar levels, as well as significantly reduced blood pressures.[1]

Don't we need the fiber that's lost in juicing?

It's true that we need to eat whole vegetables, fruit, sprouts, legumes, and whole grains for fiber. We drink juice for the extra nutrients; it's better than any vitamin pill. And for weight loss I recommend vegetable juices for appetite control. I also recommend juice as therapy. I cover more than fifty different ailments in my book *The Juice Lady's Guide to Juicing for Health* that can be improved with juice therapy, diet, and nutrients. Whole fruits and vegetables have insoluble and soluble fiber. Both types of fiber are very important for colon health. It's true that the insoluble fiber is lost when you juice. However, soluble fiber is present in juice in the form of gums and pectins. Soluble fiber is excellent for the digestive tract. It also helps to lower blood cholesterol, stabilize blood sugar, and improve good bowel bacteria. Don't worry about the fiber that is lost when you juice. Think about all the extra nutrition you are getting. Fresh juice is one of the best vitamin-mineral cocktails you could drink. You may not need as many nutritional supplements when you juice, so that could save you money in the long run. Drink your juice as a smart addition to your high-fiber diet.

Are most of the nutrients lost with the fiber?

In the past some groups have thought that a significant amount of nutrients remained in the fiber after juicing, but that theory has been disproved. The US Department of Agriculture analyzed twelve fruits and found that 90 percent of the antioxidant nutrients they measured was in the juice rather than the fiber.[2] This makes fresh juice a great supplement in the diet.

Is fresh juice better than commercially processed juice?

Fresh juice is "live food" with a full complement of vitamins, minerals, phytochemicals, and enzymes. It also contains biophotons that revitalize the body. You feel better when you drink fresh juice! In contrast, commercially processed canned, bottled, frozen, or packaged juices have been pasteurized, which means the juice has been heated and many of the vitamins and enzymes have been killed or removed. And the light energy is virtually gone. If you look at a Kirlian photograph of a cooked vegetable or a pasteurized glass of juice, you'll see very little "light" or no light emanating from them. This means the juice will have a longer shelf life, but it won't give your body life.

Making your own juice also allows you to use a wider variety of vegetables and fruit you might not otherwise eat, such as kale, beets with leaves and stems, lemon with the white part, stems, seeds, and chunks of ginger root. Some of my recipes include Jerusalem artichokes, jicama, green cabbage, celery leaves, asparagus stems, broccoli stems, kale, and parsley. These sweet, crisp tubers and healthy greens are not found in most processed juices.

How long can fresh juice be stored?

The sooner you drink fresh juice after you make it, the more nutrients you'll get. However, you can store juice and not lose too many nutrients by keeping it cold in an insulated container or covered in the refrigerator. You can also freeze it. Many busy moms are choosing to make a large batch of juice on the weekends and freeze it in individual containers.

On a personal note, when I had chronic fatigue syndrome, I would juice in the afternoons when I had the most energy and store the juice covered in the refrigerator and drink it for the next twenty-four hours until I juiced my next batch. I got well doing that.

How much produce is needed to make a glass of juice?

People often ask me if it takes a basket of produce to make a glass of juice. Actually, if you're using a good juicer, it takes a surprisingly small amount. For example, the following items yield about one 8-ounce glass of juice: five to seven large carrots or one large cucumber. The following each yield about 4 ounces of juice: one large apple, three to four large (13-inch) ribs of celery, or one large orange. The key is to get a good juicer that yields a dry pulp. I've used juicers, even expensive models, that ejected very wet pulp.

When I ran the pulp through the juicer again, I got more juice and the pulp was still wet. If the rotation speed (RPM) is too high or the juicer is not efficient in other ways, you will waste a lot of produce.

Will juicing cost lots of money?

If you were to crunch the numbers, you would find that the cost of a glass of juice is less than a latte. With three or four carrots, half a lemon, a chunk of ginger root, two ribs of celery, three or four green leaves, and half a cucumber, you will probably spend two dollars to three and a half dollars, depending on the season, the area of the country you live in, and the store where you purchase your produce. But wait—there are also hidden savings. You may not need as many vitamin supplements.

What's that worth? And you'll probably need far fewer over-the-counter medications such as painkillers; sleeping aids; antacids; laxatives; and cold, cough, and flu medications. That's a whopping savings! And then there's time not lost from work. What happens when you run out of sick days? Or if you're self-employed, you've missed out on income each day you're sick. With the immune-building, disease-fighting properties of fresh juice, you should stay well all year long.

The Basics of Juicing

Juicing is a very simple process. Simple as the procedure is, though, it helps to keep a few guidelines in mind to obtain the best results.

- *Wash all produce before juicing.* Fruit and vegetable washes are available at many grocery and health food stores. Or you can use hydrogen peroxide and then rinse. Cut away all moldy, bruised, or damaged areas of the produce.

- *Always peel oranges, tangerines, tangelos, and grapefruit* before juicing, because the skins of these citrus fruit contain volatile oils that can cause digestive problems such as stomachaches. Lemon and lime peels can be juiced, if organic, but they do add a distinct flavor that is not one of my favorites for most recipes. I usually peel them. Leave as much of the white pithy part on the citrus fruit as possible, though, since it contains the most vitamin C and bioflavonoids. Bioflavonoids work with vitamin C; they need each other to create the best uptake for your immune cells. Always peel mangoes and papayas since their skins contain an irritant that is harmful when eaten in quantity.

  I also recommend that you peel all produce that is not labeled organic even though the largest concentration of nutrients is in and next to the skin. For example, nonorganic cucumbers are often waxed, trapping the pesticides. You don't want the wax or pesticides in your juice. The peels and skins of sprayed fruits and vegetables contain the largest concentration of pesticides.

- *Remove pits, stones, and hard seeds* from fruits such as peaches, plums, apricots, cherries, and mangoes. Softer seeds from cucumbers, oranges, lemons, limes, watermelons, cantaloupes, grapes, papaya, and apples can be juiced without a problem. Because of their chemical composition, large quantities of apple seeds should not be juiced for young children under the age of two, but they should not cause problems for older children and adults.

- *The stems and leaves of most produce can be juiced.* Beet stems and leaves, strawberry caps, celery leaves, radish leaves, and small grape stems are all fine to juice, and they offer nutrients. Discard larger grape stems, as they can dull the juicer blade. Also remove carrot tops and rhubarb greens because they contain toxic substances. Cut off the ends of carrots since this is the part that molds first.

- *Cut fruits and vegetables into sections or chunks* that will fit into your juicer's feed tube. You'll learn from experience what can be added whole and what size chunks work best for your machine. If you have a large feed tube, you won't have to cut up a lot of produce.

- *Some fruits and vegetables don't juice well.* Most produce contains a lot of water, which is ideal for juicing. The vegetables and fruits that contain less water, such as bananas and avocados, will not juice well. They can be used in smoothies and cold soups by first juicing other produce, then pouring the juice into a blender and adding the avocado, for example, to make a raw soup or green smoothie. Mangoes and papayas will juice but make a thicker juice.

- *Drink your juice as soon as you can* after it's made. If you can't drink the juice right away, store it in an insulated container such as a thermos or another airtight, opaque container and in the refrigerator if possible. You can store juice for up to twenty-four hours. Light, heat, and air will destroy nutrients quickly. Be aware that the longer juice sits before you drink it, the more nutrients are lost. You can also freeze the juice. If juice turns brown, it has oxidized and lost a large amount of its nutritional value; it is not good to drink it at this point as it may be spoiled. Melon and cabbage juice do not store well; drink them soon after they've been juiced.

- When I was very sick with chronic fatigue syndrome, I had only enough energy to juice once a day. I would store some of the juice for up to twenty-four hours. I got well doing that, so I know the juice had plenty of nutrients even in the stored amount.

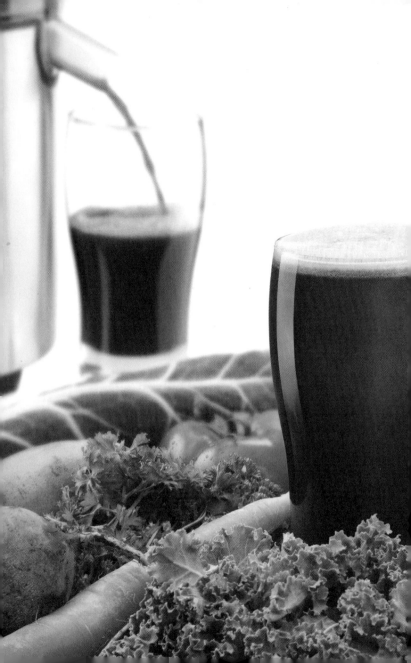

Chapter 8

LIVING FOOD, JUICE, and SMOOTHIE RECIPES THAT REDUCE STRESS and INCREASE POSITIVE ENERGY

THE RECIPES IN this chapter will help you eat meals that will assist you in managing stress and restoring your adrenal function. Keep in mind that your daily food choices make a big difference in your energy, vitality, and restoration of your body.

Living Food Recipes

Icy Spicy Gazpacho

Chili peppers actually induce the brain to secrete endorphins, those brain chemicals that are credited with the "runner's high." Endorphins block pain sensations and induce a kind of euphoria. When you're feeling great, you're less likely to go on a food binge.

2 tomatoes, cut in chunks
1 cup fresh carrot juice (about 5–7 carrots)
1 lemon, juiced, peeled if putting it through a juice machine
½ bunch cilantro, rinsed and chopped
¼ tsp. Celtic sea salt
¼ tsp. ground cumin
¼ small jalapeño, chopped (more if you like it hot)

Place the tomato chunks in a freezer bag and freeze until solid. Pour the carrot and lemon juices into a blender and add the frozen tomato chunks, cilantro, salt, cumin, and jalapeño. Blend on high speed until smooth, but slushy; serve immediately. Serves 2.

Quick Energy Soup

1 cup fresh carrot juice (5-7 medium, or approx. 1 pound, yields about 1 cup)
1 lemon, peeled if not organic
1-inch-chunk ginger root
1 avocado, peeled and seed removed
½ tsp. ground cumin

Juice the carrots, lemon, and ginger. Pour the juice in a blender. Add the avocado and cumin and blend until smooth. Serve chilled. Serves 1.

Spinach-Avocado Soup

1 cucumber, peeled, cut in chunks
1 small jalapeño, seeded
1 avocado, peeled, seed removed
Juice of 1 lemon
1–2 cloves garlic (optional)
1 Tbsp. cilantro
1 Tbsp. fresh parsley
¼ purple onion, finely chopped (for garnish)

Place all ingredients in a blender or food processor and puree until smooth. Pour into a bowl and add chopped onion, or any other chopped vegetables or herbs of choice as a garnish. Serves 2.

Summer Corn Chowder

2 cups fresh corn kernels cut off cob (about 2 large ears)
1 cup almond, oat, or rice milk
1 avocado, peeled, seed removed
¼ red bell pepper, cut in chunks
2 tsp. finely minced red onion
½ tsp. ground cumin
½ tsp. Celtic sea salt
Garnish: 1 Tbsp. each, chopped parsley and minced red bell pepper
   (optional)

In a blender, combine the corn, milk, avocado, bell pepper, onion, cumin, and salt. Blender well. Pour into bowls and garnish with parsley and red pepper. Serves 2.

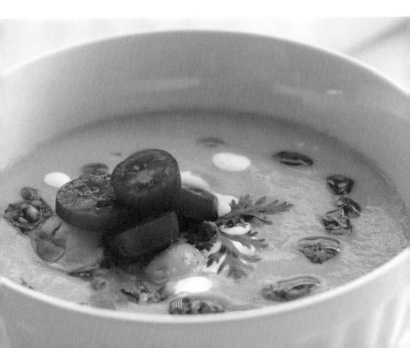

Creamy Tomato Soup

1–2 tomatoes
1 avocado, peeled, seed removed
2 Tbsp. chopped sweet red bell pepper
¼ carrot, chopped in small pieces
½ cup rice, oat, or almond milk

Combine all ingredients in a blender and blend well. Pour into bowls. Serves 2.

Refreshing Cucumber-Mint Soup

1 cucumber, peeled if not organic and cut into chunks
1 avocado, peeled, seed removed
¼–½ cup chopped fresh mint

Combine all ingredients in a blender and blend well. Pour into a bowl. Serves 1.

French Tomato Basil Soup

3 medium tomatoes
Juice of 1 lemon
1 avocado, peeled, seed removed
2 Tbsp. chopped fresh basil
1 small garlic clove
Fresh basil leaves chopped for garnish (optional)

In a blender, blend the tomatoes until chunky. Add the lemon, avocado, basil, and garlic. Blend well. Pour into bowls and garnish with fresh basil leaves, as desired. Serves 2.

Kale Spinach Soup

3 large kale leaves
3 stalks celery
1 lemon, peeled if not organic
1 avocado, peeled, seed removed
1 cup spinach leaves

Juice the kale, celery, and lemon. Pour into a blender, add the avocado and spinach, and blend well. Pour into bowls and serve. Serves 2.

Tomato Asparagus Soup

10 stalks asparagus, chopped
4 tomatoes, cut in chunks
3–4 sun-dried tomatoes
2 cloves garlic
¼ cup fresh parsley, chopped
¼ cup lemon juice
½ red bell pepper, chopped
1 tsp. Celtic sea salt
1 avocado, peeled, seed removed

Combine asparagus, tomatoes, sun-dried tomatoes, garlic, parsley, lemon juice, bell pepper, and salt in a blender and blend well. Add the avocado and blend well. Pour into bowls and serve. Serves 2.

Cucumber Dill Soup

1¼ cups fresh cucumber juice (about 1 large or 2 medium cucumbers, peeled if not organic)
2 stalks celery with leaves, juiced
1 avocado, peeled, seed removed
1 garlic clove, peeled
½ cup almond, oat, or rice milk
½ cup parsley, coarsely chopped
2 tsp. red onion, chopped
3 tsp. fresh dill weed or 1–2 tsp. dried

Pour the cucumber and celery juices into a blender and add the avocado, garlic, milk, parsley, onion, and dill. Blend on high speed until smooth and serve immediately. This soup is not good if it sits. Serves 2.

Dehydrated Foods

Dehydrated foods make great snacks that can help you lose weight much more easily because they offer taste satisfaction without a lot of calories. For example, Kale Chips are very low in calories and exceptionally high in nutrients such as calcium, magnesium, and vitamin K. Onion Rings, Dehydrated Tomatoes, Garlicky Jicama Crackers, and Dehydrated Zucchini make wonderful snacks or accompaniment to meals and offer bursts of flavor along with fiber, enzymes, and a cornucopia of nutrients. It doesn't take much time to prepare them and the rewards are great.

You'll notice that the dehydration temperature varies in all the recipes between 105 and 115 degrees Fahrenheit. There are a number of schools of thought as to what the best temperature is to preserve the most enzymes and vitamins. When in doubt, choose the lower temperature setting on your dehydrator.

Kale Chips

1 bunch kale
¼ cup apple cider or coconut vinegar
¼ cup fresh lemon juice
¼ cup extra-virgin olive oil
½ tsp. Celtic sea salt
2 tsp. garlic, minced or pressed (optional)
Pinch of cayenne pepper

Wash the kale and then cut it into 3-inch long strips and set aside to dry. Add vinegar and lemon juice to a bowl. Very slowly, pour in the olive oil by dripping it in from a distance of about a foot above the bowl while whisking continually. This will create an emulsion where the oil is well combined with the other ingredients and won't separate as easily so you won't end up with lots of oil on some pieces and very little on others. Then stir in the sea salt, minced garlic, if using, and cayenne. Shake off excess marinade and place kale pieces on dehydrator sheets and dehydrate for about 7 to 8 hours at 105 to 115 degrees Fahrenheit or until crisp. (Chips will get smaller as they dehydrate.)

These chips are so delicious I'll bet you won't have any left to store. Makes about 4 trays of chips.

Dehydrated Zucchini Chips

Slice zucchini into thin rounds and sprinkle with a little Celtic sea salt, as desired. You can also sprinkle your favorite seasoning on them. Place zucchini slices on dehydrator sheets and dehydrate for about 12 hours at 105 to 115 degrees Fahrenheit or until crispy. They are surprisingly sweet and delicious.

Onion Rings

3–5 onions (yellow, white, Walla Walla sweets)
¼ cup apple cider or coconut vinegar
¼ cup fresh lemon juice
¼ cup extra-virgin olive oil
½ tsp. Celtic sea salt
2 tsp. garlic, minced or pressed, optional
Pinch of cayenne pepper

Cut onions into thin slices and set aside. Add vinegar and lemon juice to a bowl. Very slowly, pour in the olive oil by dripping it in from a distance of about a foot above the bowl while whisking continually. This will create an emulsion where the oil is well combined with the other ingredients and won't separate as easily so you won't end up with lots of oil on some pieces and very little on others. Then stir in the sea salt, minced garlic, if using, and cayenne. Add the onion slices to the emulsion and marinate for several hours. Shake off excess marinade so that onion rings are not dripping with marinate. Place onions rings on dehydrator sheets and dehydrate for about 7 to 8 hours at 105 to 115 degrees Fahrenheit or until crisp.

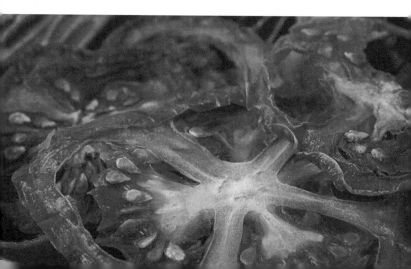

Dehydrated Tomatoes and Basil

Slice tomatoes thinly and put a fresh basil leaf on top of each slice, once you've placed them on a dehydrator sheet. Dehydrate for about 12 hours at 105 to 115 degrees Fahrenheit or until crispy.

Flax Crackers

Flaxseeds are rich in alpha-linolenic acid (ALA)—a type of plant-derived omega-3 fatty acid, similar to those found in fish such as salmon. Benefits of flaxseed as shown in many studies include lowering LDL cholesterol. Other benefits show that flaxseeds may help lower blood triglycerides and blood pressure. It may also keep platelets from becoming sticky, therefore reducing the risk of a heart attack.

2 cups flaxseeds
1 red bell pepper
1 carrot
½ cup sun-dried tomatoes
2 cups fresh tomatoes
Juice of 1 lemon
1 clove of fresh garlic
1 Tbsp. shoyu, tamari, or Braggs liquid aminos or 1–2 tsp. Celtic sea salt

Blend all ingredients together in a food processor. Add water if the batter is too dry. Press mixture flat onto a P-Flexx sheet into a large square that covers the sheet. Make sure that the mixture stands only about ⅛-inch high. The thicker the cracker, the chewier it is and the longer it takes to dry. With a knife or spatula, score the batch to the size you'd like before dehydrating. (A typical square is 3x3.) Dehydrate around 105 degrees Fahrenheit overnight; flip over once one side is dry. Dehydrate until completely dry. Store in an airtight container. Makes about 27 crackers.

Broccoli Latkes

1½ pounds of broccoli (you can use the stems)
½ pound of daikon radish
1 medium onion, cut into chunks
1 cup tahini
1 tsp. Celtic sea salt
½ tsp. black pepper

Place broccoli and daikon radish in the food processor and process until shredded. Scoop this mixture into a bowl. Add the chunks of onion to the food processor and process until in small pieces; add to the bowl. Blend together the tahini, salt, and pepper. Add this mixture to the vegetables in the bowl and mix well with your hands. Form into patties about 3 inches in diameter on dehydrator sheets. Dehydrate 8–10 hours and then turn them over carefully. Dehydrate another 8–10 hours or until completely dry. Makes about 27 crackers.

Garlicky Jicama Crackers

1 tomato, diced
1 red or yellow bell pepper, minced
1 tsp. Celtic sea salt
¼ cup extra-virgin olive oil
8–10 cloves of garlic, minced or pressed
1 tsp. fresh oregano, finely chopped or ½ tsp. dried
1 tsp. fresh basil, finely chopped or ½ tsp. dried
1 medium jicama, thinly sliced

Combine all ingredients except the jicama in a bowl and mix well. Arrange jicama slices on a dehydrator sheet. Spoon about 1 teaspoon of the tomato mixture onto each jicama slice and spread evenly. Dehydrate for about 24 hours at 105 to 115 degrees Fahrenheit or until the jicama cracker is crisp. (Jicama will curl at edges.) Makes 12–15 crackers.

Veggie Crackers

1 onion, chopped
2 celery stalks, chopped
1 yellow or red bell pepper, chopped
1 tomato, chopped
1 large carrot, chopped
½ cup green peas
½ cup fresh corn cut from cob, or frozen
½ cup sesame seeds, soaked for several hours

Place all ingredients in a food processor and blend until slightly chunky. Spread on dehydrator sheets and dehydrate for 12 to 20 hours at at 105 to 115 degrees Fahrenheit or until crispy. Makes about 15 crackers.

Seed Crackers

1 cup flaxseeds soaked in 2 cups purified water overnight
1 cup sunflower seeds soaked overnight
1 cup almonds soaked overnight
1 cup yellow bell pepper, chopped
1 cup yellow squash, chopped
½ cup celery, chopped
3 Tbsp. fresh oregano or 1½ Tbsp. dried
1 Tbsp. onion powder
2 tsp. Celtic sea salt

Blend flaxseeds, sunflower seeds, and nuts in a food processor until smooth. Add the other ingredients and process until smooth. Spread in thin layer on a dehydrator sheet and dehydrate for 12 to 20 hours at 105 to 115 degrees Fahrenheit until crisp. Makes about 36 crackers.

Guilt-Free "Bacon"

¼ cup extra-virgin olive oil
4 Tbsp. apple cider vinegar
2 Tbsp. honey
1 tsp. ground black pepper
1 eggplant, thinly sliced into strips

Mix together the olive oil, vinegar, honey and pepper, and marinate the eggplant strips for at least 2 hours in the mixture. Then place the strips on a dehydrator sheet and dehydrate for 12 hours at 105 to 115 degrees Fahrenheit. Turn strips over and dehydrate another 12 hours.

Main Course Raw Vegan

Asian Salad

2 zucchini, sliced into strips with a vegetable peeler or mandolin
2 large handfuls of bean sprouts, approx. 2 cups
¾ cup chopped nuts (use almonds or cashews)
1 red or yellow bell pepper, sliced into strips
4 green onions, diced
½ cup fresh chopped cilantro
Juice from one lime
1 Tbsp. extra-virgin olive oil
½ tsp. Celtic sea salt

Toss all ingredients together in a bowl until well coated.

South-of-the Border Lettuce Wraps

2 ripe avocados
3 tomatoes, diced

½ jalapeño pepper, diced
2 Tbsp. yellow onion, diced
3 cloves fresh garlic, minced
¼ cup fresh cilantro, chopped
Kernels cut from one ear raw corn
2 tsp. fresh lime juice
6–8 large lettuce leaves

In a medium sized bowl, mash the avocados. Add the remaining ingredients and stir until well mixed. Spread 2–3 tablespoons of this mixture onto lettuce leaves and wrap. Serves 6–8.

Jalapeño Nut Burgers

1 cup walnuts, soaked for 4 hours
¼ cup sun-dried tomatoes, soaked until very soft, reserve ⅛ cup
    soaking water
1 jalapeño pepper, finely chopped
½ onion, finely chopped
1 tsp. Celtic sea salt
1 tsp. hamburger seasoning
½ tsp. black pepper

In a food processor, combine walnuts, sun-dried tomatoes, and soaking water until you achieve a meat consistency. Remove from processor. Place the nut mixture in a bowl, and combine with the jalapeño pepper, onions, seasoning, salt, and pepper. Shape into 6 patties. Dehydrate at 105 to 115 degrees Fahrenheit degrees for 3 to 4 hours. Serves 6.

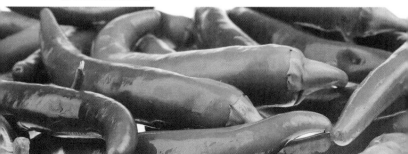

Stuffed Bell Peppers

6 medium carrots, chopped
1–2 celery stalks, chopped
1 large or 2 small ripe avocados
1 tsp. dulse or Celtic sea salt
½ cup chopped cucumber
½ cup chopped tomato
½ tsp. cumin
1 large red or yellow bell pepper
Raw sunflower seeds for garnish

Place carrots and celery in a food processor and process until pulp consistency, or use carrot and celery pulp leftover from juicing. Transfer the pulp to a bowl. Remove the flesh from the avocado(s) and, using a fork, mash the avocado into the carrot-clery pulp. Add the dulse or salt, cucumber, tomato, and cumin and mix well. Cut bell pepper in half; scoop out the seeds, and stuff with the carrot-avocado mixture. Top each stuffed pepper with a teaspoon of sunflower seeds. Serves 2.

Spicy Peanut Sauce Over Zucchini Noodles

½ cup raw peanut butter or almond butter
1–2 tsp. hot chili oil
2–3 tsp. tamari, Nama Shoyu, or organic soy sauce
1 clove minced garlic
1 tsp. virgin coconut oil
2–3 yellow summer squash or zucchini, made into noodles

In a food processor combine everything except the coconut oil and squash noodles. until well blended. Add the oil just until the sauce is of the consistency you like. Adjust tamari, shoyu or soy sauce and chili oil to taste.

This sauce tastes fantastic, and if you let it sit a bit, it gets even better.

Serve it over summer squash or zucchini noodles made with spiral slicer or spirooli slicer. Yellow summer squash is a bit sturdier than zucchini and works well with the spicy peanut sauce. Serves 4.

Easy Phad Thai

3 zucchini, processed into noodles with a spiral slicer or spirooli slicer
1 package (3½ oz.) enoki mushrooms, trimmed and separated
3 green onions, thinly sliced
1 red bell pepper, cut into thin strips
10 snow peas
½ pound mung bean sprouts
½ lime, juiced
½ tsp. Celtic sea salt
1 Tbsp. extra-virgin olive oil

Topping

1 cup almonds, chopped
½ cup cilantro, chopped
Handful bean sprouts

In a bowl, combine all the ingredients except for the topping ingredients and stir well. Spoon Phad Thai Sauce over top and sprinkle topping over sauce.

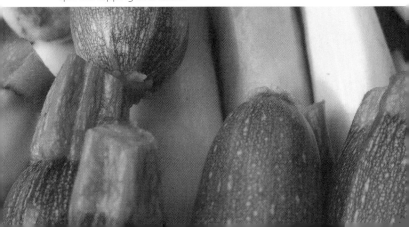

Phad Thai Sauce

1 Tbsp. hiziki seaweed soaked for 30 minutes or more in enough water
    to cover (optional)
½ cup raw almond butter
½ cup sun-dried tomatoes, soaked 2 hours
1 lime, chopped (including peel if organic)
4 garlic cloves, peeled and finely chopped or pressed
7 dates, pitted and chopped
½ cup extra-virgin olive oil
2 small Thai chilies or 1 jalapeño (do not remove seeds if you like it hot)
1½ Tbsp. grated fresh ginger
1–2 Tbsp. tamari, plus extra if desired or 1 tsp. Celtic sea salt
½ cup purified water
1 cup cilantro, loosely packed, chopped
Juice of ½ lemon or line or about 1½ Tbsp.
1 Tbsp. maple syrup or date paste

Blend the hiziki, if using, almond butter, sun-dried tomatoes, lime, garlic, dates, olive oil, chilies, ginger, and tamari or sea salt with ½ cup water until creamy. Add additional ingredients and blend again.

Gourmet Raw Pizza

(This is a higher calorie recipe that should be enjoyed after you've reached your weight loss goal.)

Raw Buckwheat Groat Pizza Dough

This recipe also makes a delicious Italian Buckwheat cracker.

2 cups sprouted buckwheat groats*

---

* To sprout buckwheat, soak 1 cup raw buckwheat groats for about 2 hours; it will expand to about 2 cups. Drain and rinse well. Place on counter in a colander covered with a light-weight dishtowel or sprouter for one day. Rinse several times while sprouting. (If you don't have time to sprout, you can use buckwheat that has been soaked for 2 hours.)

1–2 garlic cloves, chopped
¾ cup finely grated carrots (or use carrot pulp)
¾ cup soaked flaxseeds (soak overnight; they'll expand to about 1½
    cups, or use ground flaxseeds and extra water)
½ cup extra-virgin olive oil
1 Tbsp. Italian seasonings (or fresh herbs to taste)
1–2 tsp. Celtic sea salt
Water as needed (usually ½–1 cup)

Mix all ingredients together in a food processor. Start with buckwheat groats and garlic followed by the rest of the ingredients. Coat a dehydrator sheet sheet with a small amount of olive oil and scoop batches of dough (about a heaping tablespoon each) onto dehydrator sheets and swirl each scoop with a spoon to make rounds. You can make large pizza dough (about 6 inches in diameter)—or you can make smaller individual rounds (about 3 inches in diameter). The smaller rounds are easier to serve and eat. Press out the dough evenly to about ⅛ to ¼ inch thick by patting the top with your fingertips or swirling with a spoon. If it gets too sticky, dip your fingers into some water to which you add a little olive oil. Once crust is pressed out evenly, dehydrate at 105–115 degrees Fahrenheit for about 7 hours. Flip the crackers and dry another 7 to 10 hours or until crust is completely dry and crisp. (It should be crunchy for the best tasting cracker.) To speed the drying process, transfer to the mesh rack. Use a spatula when lifting dough and be careful when transferring it not to break the crackers.

   NOTE: If crust is very dry, and stored in a cool dry, airtight container, it can be kept fresh for several months.

Nutty Cheese Sauce for Pizza Topping

1 cup macadamia nuts and 1 cup raw pine nuts, soaked or 2 cups
     cashews, soaked (cashews are a bit sweeter and usually less
     expensive)
½ cup lemon juice
1½ tsp. Celtic sea salt
1 Tbsp. garlic, chopped
½ tsp. peppercorns (ground)
Water as needed

Soak nuts first for several hours. Blend all ingredients until very
creamy. Blend for about 3 to 4 minutes for the creamiest sauce. Add
water as needed. This sauce will keep 3 days in the refrigerator in a
covered container.

Yummy Marinara Sauce

This sauce is also great on raw spaghetti.

½ cup dried pineapple, soaked (or fresh)
2 cups chopped tomatoes
1 tsp. ginger, minced
2 Tbsp. garlic, minced
1 tsp. jalapeño, minced
⅓ cup fresh basil leaves, chopped and packed or 2 tablespoons dried
¼ cup red bell pepper, chopped
⅓ cup sun-dried tomatoes, soaked
⅓ cup fresh oregano leaves-de-stemmed and chopped, or 2
     tablespoons dried
¼ cup Nama Shoyu or 1½ teaspoons Celtic sea salt
1 cup extra virgin olive oil

Blend all ingredients together in a food processor. If it the sauce sets
in the refrigerator for at least an hour, it will thicken and become
more flavorful.
     To assemble pizza: Arrange buckwheat pizza crackers on a plate.

Spoon about 2 teaspoons of the marinara sauce on the top of each cracker. It should be thick and not run over the edges. Top with several little dollops of Nutty Cheese Sauce. If the Nutty Cheese Sauce is too thick, add a little water. It should still be thick and not at all runny. Place about ½ teaspoon of cheese sauce in a few places on top of the marinara sauce. For a garnish, top pizza with finely chopped scallions, onions, black olives, or leeks.

Juice Recipes

Waldorf Morning

1 green apple
3 ribs of celery with leaves
1 lemon, peeled if not organic
½ cucumber, peeled if not organic

Cut produce to fit your juicer's feed tube. Juice ingredients and stir. Pour into a glass and drink as soon as possible. Serves 1.

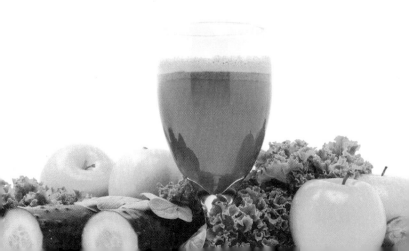

Cherie's Morning Blend

Rather than coffee, why not wake up your body with an energizing, delicious juice?

4–5 carrots, scrubbed well, tops removed, ends trimmed
4 dark green leaves, such as chard, kale, or collards
2 ribs of celery with leaves
1 large cucumber, peeled if not organic
1 lemon peeled, if not organic
1-inch-chunk ginger root

Cut produce to fit your juicer's feed tube. Juice ingredients and stir. Pour into a glass and drink as soon as possible. Serves 2.

Cool Cucumber

1 cucumber, peeled if not organic
2 ribs of celery with leaves
2 leaves baby bok choy
2 romaine lettuce leaves
2–3 carrots, scrubbed well, tops removed, ends trimmed
3–4 sprigs cilantro
3–4 sprigs mint
1 lime, peeled if not organic

Cut produce to fit your juicer's feed tube. Juice all ingredients, stir, and drink as soon as possible. Serves 2.

Magnesium Special

4–5 beet tops
2 Swiss chard leaves
2 collard leaves
1 cucumber, peeled if not organic
½ green apple (omit if diabetic)
½ lemon, peeled if not organic

Cut produce to fit your juicer's feed tube. Juice ingredients and stir.
Pour into a glass and drink as soon as possible. Serves 2.

Energize-Your-Day Cocktail

1 apple (green is lower in sugar)
2 dark green leaves (chard, collard, or kale)
1 rib of celery with leaves
1 lemon, peeled if not organic
½ cucumber, peeled if not organic
½ - to 1-inch-chunk fresh ginger root, peeled

Cut the apple into sections that fit your juicer's
feed tube. Roll the green leaves and push through
the feed tube with the apple, celery, lemon,
cucumber, and ginger. Stir the juice and pour into
a glass. Drink as soon as possible. Serves 1.

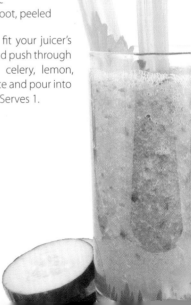

Happy-Mood Morning

Fennel juice has been used as a traditional tonic to help the body release endorphins, the "feel-good" peptides, from the brain into the bloodstream. Endorphins help to diminish anxiety and fear, and they generate a mood of euphoria.

½ apple (green is lower in sugar)
4–5 carrots, well scrubbed, tops removed, ends trimmed
3 fennel stalks with leaves and flowers
½ cucumber, peeled if not organic
1 handful of spinach
1-inch-chunk ginger root

Cut produce to fit your juicer's feed tube. Juice apple first and follow with other ingredients. Stir and pour into a glass; drink as soon as possible. Serves 1–2.

Adrenal Booster

Hot peppers and parsley are rich in vitamin C; celery is a great source of natural sodium. Both are very beneficial for the adrenal glands.

1 handful of parsley
1 dark green lettuce leaf
4 carrots, scrubbed well, tops removed, ends trimmed
2 tomatoes
2 ribs of celery with leaves
Dash of hot sauce
Dash of Celtic sea salt

Cut produce to fit your juicer's feed tube. Wrap the parsley in the lettuce leaf and push through the juicer slowly. Juice all remaining ingredients, add hot sauce and sea salt, and stir. Pour into a glass and drink as soon as possible. Serves 2.

Antianxiety Cocktail

As I stated in chapter 6, magnesium is known as "nature's Valium." If you're prone to anxiety attacks, include plenty of magnesium-rich veggies such as beet leaves, spinach, parsley, dandelion greens, broccoli, cauliflower, carrots, and celery in your juices.

3–4 carrots, scrubbed well, tops removed, ends trimmed
2 ribs of celery with leaves
1 handful of spinach
1 dark green lettuce leaf
1 broccoli stem
1 lemon, peeled if not organic

Cut produce to fit your juicer's feed tube. Juice all ingredients and stir. Pour into a glass and drink as soon as possible. Serves 1.

Magnesium Cocktail

The American diet is very low in magnesium. One of magnesium's most important benefits is that it lowers the risk of cardiovascular disease. It's also very helpful for depression, insomnia, and migraines. Juice up plenty of magnesium-rich greens such as beet greens, spinach, chard, collards, parsley, and dandelion greens.

1 handful of parsley
3–4 leaves of chard or collards
3–4 carrots, scrubbed well, tops removed, ends trimmed
2 ribs of celery, with leaves as desired
½ small beet with leaves
1 lemon, peeled if not organic

Cut produce to fit your juicer's feed tube. Wrap parsley in the green leaves and push through the juicer slowly. Juice all remaining ingredients and stir. Pour into a glass and drink as soon as possible. Serves 1.

Mood Mender Tonic

Antidepressant use has been linked to thicker arteries, which could contribute to the risk of heart disease and stroke. Raise your endorphins naturally with foods such as fennel. Fennel juice has been used as a traditional remedy to help the body release endorphins into the bloodstream. Endorphins are the "feel-good" peptides from the brain that help to diminish anxiety and fear and generate a mood of euphoria.

3 fennel stalks with bulbs and fronds
3–4 carrots, scrubbed well, tops removed, ends trimmed
2 ribs of celery with leaves
½ pear or ½ apple
½ lemon, peeled if not organic
1-inch-chunk ginger root, peeled

Cut produce to fit your juicer's feed tube. Juice ingredients and stir. Pour into glasses and drink as soon as possible. Serves 2.

Sleep Rejuvenator

Celery has a calming effect, and lettuce is a natural sedative.

2 romaine lettuce leaves
2 ribs of celery with leaves
1 lemon, peeled if not organic
5 medium carrots, scrubbed well, tops removed, ends trimmed
4 cauliflower florets, washed

Cut produce to fit your juicer's feed tube. Juice ingredients and stir. Pour into a glass and drink as soon as possible. Serves 1.

Green Recharger

1 cucumber, peeled if not organic
1 handful sunflower sprouts
1 handful buckwheat sprouts
1 small handful clover sprouts
1 kale leaf
1 large handful spinach
1 lime, peeled if not organic

Cut the cucumber to fit your juicer's feed tube. Juice half of the
cucumber first. Bunch up the sprouts and wrap in the kale leaf.
Turn off the machine and add them. Turn the machine back on and
tap with the rest of the cucumber to gently push the sprouts and
kale through followed by the spinach. Then juice the remaining
cucumber and lime. Stir ingredients, pour into a glass, and drink as
soon as possible. Serves 1–2.

Wild Green Energy Cocktail

Wild greens reduce the desire for starchy foods, thus making them
an excellent weight-loss helper.

1 cucumber, peeled if not organic
1 celery stalk
1 handful wild greens such as
    dandelion, nettles, plantain, lamb's
    quarters, or sorrel
1 apple (green is lower in sugar)
1 lemon, peeled if not organic

Cut all ingredients to fit your juicer's feed tube. Juice all ingredients
and stir. Pour into a glass and drink as soon as possible. Serves 1.

The Morning Energizer

4 carrots, scrubbed well, green tops removed, ends trimmed
1 handful parsley
1 lemon, peeled if not organic
1 apple (green has less sugar)
2-inch-chunk fresh ginger root, peeled

Cut produce to fit your juicer's feed tube. Juice all ingredients and stir. Pour into a glass and drink as soon as possible. Serves 1.

Energize-Your-Day Cocktail

1 apple (green is lower in sugar)
2 dark green leaves (chard, collard, or kale)
1 stalk celery with leaves
1 lemon, peeled if not organic
½ cucumber, peeled if not organic
½- to 1-inch-chunk fresh ginger root, peeled

Cut the apple into sections that fit your juicer's feed tube. Roll the green leaves and push through the feed tube with the apple, celery, lemon, cucumber, and ginger. Stir the juice and pour into a glass. Drink as soon as possible. Serves 1.

Vitamin C–Rich Combinations

Vitamin C is important for healthy adrenal glands and immune system that chronic stress can sometimes break down, detoxification, eyes, collagen, bone structure, cartilage, muscle, veins, capillaries, teeth, and gums. The richest sources of vitamin C include chili peppers, kale, parsley, collard greens, turnip greens, broccoli, mustard greens, watercress, spinach, lemon, and Swiss chard.

Carrot and Spice

2–3 carrots, scrubbed well, tops removed, ends trimmed
1 handful spinach
1 cucumber, peeled if not organic
½ lemon, peeled if not organic
½ apple (green has less sugar)
1-inch-chunk ginger root
¼ tsp. cinnamon
⅛ tsp. cayenne pepper

Cut produce to fit your juicer's feed tube. Juice all ingredients
except spices. Pour juice into a glass, add spices, stir, and drink as
soon as possible. Serves 2.

Raging Beet-Jalapeño

1 beet with tops
2 collard or Swiss chard leaves
1 cucumber, peeled if not organic
1 lemon, peeled if not organic
1-inch-chunk ginger root
½ small jalapeño, seeds removed

Cut produce to fit your juicer's feed tube. Juice the beet with its
tops. Roll collard or chard leaves and follow with ½ cucumber. Add
other ingredients and follow with the remaining cucumber. Pour
juice into a glass, stir, and drink as soon as possible. Serves 1.

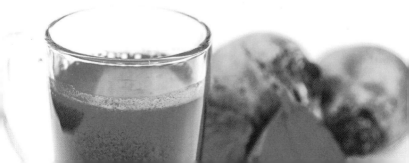

Peppy Parsley

1 cucumber, peeled if not organic
1 carrot, scrubbed well, green tops removed, ends trimmed
1 stalk celery with leaves
1 handful parsley
1 kale leaf
1 lemon, peeled if not organic

Cut produce to fit your juicer's feed tube. Juice the cucumber, carrot, and celery. Bunch up parsley and roll in kale leaf; add to juicer and push through. Then add lemon and juice. Stir and pour into a glass. Drink as soon as possible. Serves 1.

Triple C Ulcer Mender

Scientific research has proven that cabbage juice is an effective treatment for stomach ulcers.[1] By itself it does not taste good, but with about equal parts of carrot and celery, it has a slightly nutty taste. (Avoid citrus if you have an ulcer; they can aggravate symptoms.)

¼ small head green cabbage
3 carrots, scrubbed well, tops removed, ends trimmed
4 celery stalks, with leaves if desired

Cut produce to fit your juicer's feed tube. Juice all ingredients and stir. You will need to drink this right away as cabbage juice does not store well. Serves 1.

Cabbage Patch (Ulcer Healer)

Sulforaphane is a compound in cabbage, broccoli, cauliflower, and kale that has been reported to inhibit antibiotic-resistant strains of *Helicobacter pylori* (which cause ulcers). Broccoli sprouts contain from thirty to fifty times the concentration of this chemical as in the mature plants. This effect was identified by scientists at the Johns Hopkins University School of Medicine in Baltimore while investigating sulforaphane for its protective effect against cancer.[2]

3 stalks celery with leaves
3 carrots, scrubbed well, tops removed, ends trimmed
1 cucumber, peeled if not organic
1 lemon, peeled if not organic
¼ green cabbage (spring or summer cabbage is best)
Handful broccoli sprouts (optional)

Cut produce to fit your juicer's feed tube. Juice all ingredients and stir. Pour into a glass and drink as soon as possible. Serves 1.

The Pink Onion (Stomach Cancer and Ulcer Fighter)

The odorous sulfur compounds found in onions help fight the *H. pylori* bacteria, which is linked with ulcers and stomach cancer.

3 carrots, scrubbed well, tops removed, ends trimmed
2 stalks celery
1 small beet with tops
1 cucumber, peeled if not organic
½ sweet onion
½ pear

Cut produce to fit your juicer's feed tube. Juice all ingredients and stir. Pour into a glass and drink as soon as possible. Serves 2.

Sweet Sleep Cocktail

Lettuce and celery help the body relax and help you sleep more deeply.

5 medium carrots, scrubbed well, green tops removed, ends trimmed
2 stalks celery
2 romaine lettuce leaves
1 kale leaf
1 lemon, peeled if not organic
½ green apple, optional

Cut produce to fit your juicer's feed tube. Juice all ingredients and stir. Pour into a glass and drink as soon as possible. Serves 1.

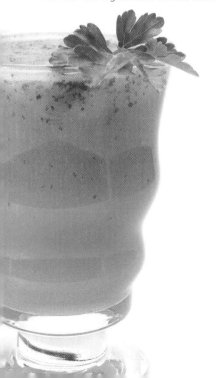

Conclusion

A STRESS-FREE FUTURE IS YOURS for the TAKING

WHILE WE CAN'T always control the things that happen to us from day to day, we can control how we respond to them. Making healthy choices for your mind, body, and spirit can limit the negative and toxic effects certain stressors have on you. Living a healthy lifestyle and having a well-balanced plan in place will put you ahead of the curve. This is being proactive rather than reactive. Stress intensifies when you feel you have no control over what is going on. However, believing you don't have control may be more perception than reality. You have the power to change the way you see your life right now. You can stop where you are, stop rehearsing the what-ifs or could-haves of the past, and set yourself on the right path to peace and wellness.

The choices you make today will create the person you want to be in the future. Taking action is key. If you continue in the same old rut, you will get more of the same, and nothing will change. It's time to get going on a new plan of action. Research indicates that people who have active and balanced lifestyles appear to have what can be called a "compelling future." This means that having a picture of a positive future can motivate you to do what is necessary to make your desired future a reality.

Here's what you can do right now. Imagine yourself six months to a year from now. We'll call this your "future self." When you see your future self clearly, imagine moving over and physically becoming that person. Now step back and look at your future self again. Ask that future self what he or she wants you to begin doing now to have a more peaceful, balanced, stress-free, and healthy lifestyle that can create that future desired self. Whatever your future self says, write it down. Take a look around you. Notice several people who are older than you. Think about them one at a time. Which one is most like the person you'd like to be five, ten, fifteen, and twenty years from now? Which one is closest to living the lifestyle that you would like to have at that age? Write down the activities and health habits that person has developed.

Remember that each day you are creating one of two pictures—your best or your worst self. People who create the best possible future make continual positive decisions for health's sake, such as juicing vegetables each day and exercising thirty minutes to an hour, three or four times a week. They often use the stairs rather than an elevator and order more salads than sandwiches or pizza. They take more walks. They spend more time in positive pursuits. And they know about deferred gratification. They think about the consequences of daily decisions and how these choices steer them away from or toward their best future self.

Now cut out or draw a picture of your best future self and one of your worst future self. Underneath each picture write down the good or bad habits that would create either person. Put these pictures up where you can look at them every day. Each morning make a decision to choose activities and actions that will correspond with creating your best self. The rewards are immense. It's worth the effort. Every evening look again at the two pictures and evaluate which picture you moved toward that day by your actions.

This isn't an exercise in futility or someone's gimmicky idea that doesn't change a thing. Writing down goals and making collages really do work. It's worked over and over again for me.

Take time to seriously think about what kind of body you will need to complete your goals and dreams. What weight should you be at to meet your goals? What level of mental and emotional health do you need to be at to fulfill your destiny?

Your future is in your hands—one choice, maybe one sip of juice or bite of food at a time.

You Have a Purpose

After all that happened to me, including dying and coming back, I knew there was a purpose for my life—a reason I had lived. I could help others find their way to wholeness—body, soul, and spirit. I could help people—maybe you—let go of emotional pain, stress, and anxiety and make healthy choices for life.

There's a purpose for your life. All the pain, trauma, rejection, disappointment, or loss you've experienced can become the fabric of your stronger soul and the launching pad for a life lived to the fullest. You can reach out to the world with a generous heart and make a difference right where you live and around the world, if that's your goal.

A number of years ago when I was on air on QVC as spokesperson for the George Foreman grills, one of the men in the maintenance department at the hotel where I stayed would drive me in the hotel van to QVC for evening shows. We'd talk about our lives on the way. He may have been a maintenance man by night, but by day he had a special purpose in his neighborhood. Many of the single parents worked long hours. Because he worked the late-night shift at the hotel, he had time to give to neighborhood kids in the afternoon. He and his wife and their children opened their home after school to the kids who had nowhere to go. He'd barbecue for them, play games with them, take them to ball games, and out on Saturday fishing trips in the summer. He gave those kids many happy memories where they would have otherwise been lonely kids maybe getting in trouble after school. Who knows what kinds of problems he saved those kids from experiencing because he was there living his purpose?

Often, as this man related stories of the kids to me, I'd think about purpose. He made me so aware that each of us has a purpose, a place we can make a difference in this world. What's yours? Have you discovered it yet? I'm sure you have more than one purpose—and being too exhausted and stressed to be of any good is not one of them.

Why should you work hard to stay at the top of your physical game? Why not succumb to momentary pleasures like grabbing a bag of chips and polishing them off? Or buying a box of Milk Duds for the movie? There's a bigger picture for your life than just getting through a day. You need a healthy, fit, strong body to complete your goals. The temporary "fixes," those little food addictions and cravings that many of us wink at, could be keeping you from the great joy of fulfilling the reason you're here on this earth. There are people waiting for you—*just you*. Nobody else can do what you do.

When you discover and fully embrace your purpose, you will be able to more fully embrace a healthy way of life and let go of the foods and behaviors that don't serve you well. If you're clueless as to what your purpose is, pray. That's what I did each time I made a future list or a collage of pictures.

Why not do what I did? Make a storyboard. Cut out pictures from magazines that represent goals you want to achieve, dreams you want to fulfill, and people you want to help. Make it a prayer walk into the future. Paste a representation of everything you want to fulfill onto that blank sheet of paper. Put it up where you can see it often. I had mine posted on the inside door of my desk. I looked at it each time I reached for office supplies. Everything on that storyboard has come true but one thing.

In the meantime get ready physically. You need energy, a fit body, clear mind, and abundant health to complete your goals. You can choose today to live healthy, fit, and strong so you can share your gifts with the world and fulfill your purpose.

NOTES

Chapter 2—You Can't Control Everything

1. Melinda Beck, "Putting an End to Mindless Munching," *Wall Street Journal*, May 13, 2008, http://online.wsj.com/article/SB12106298537798635l.html (accessed August 2, 2013).

Chapter 3—Chronic Stress and Adrenal Fatigue

1. James Wilson, "Chronic Fatigue Syndrome," AdrenalFatigue.org, http://www.adrenalfatigue.org/chronic-fatigue-syndrome (accessed August 5, 2013). Used by permission.

2. Christiane Northrup, "Adrenal Exhaustion," DrNorthrup.com, http://www.drnorthrup.com/womenshealth/healthcenter/topic_details.php?topic_id=94 (accessed August 23, 2013).

3. Ibid.

Chapter 4—Living Foods Increase Vitality and Inner Peace

1. Joseph Mercola, "McDonald's and Biophoton Deficiency," Mercola.com, August 21, 2002, http://articles.mercola.com/sites/articles/archive/2002/08/21/biophoton.aspx (accessed August 5, 2013).

2. John Switzer, "Bio-Photon Nutrition and Wild Green Energy Cocktails for Optimal Health (English)," May 21, 2009, http://tinyurl.com/nrtvvsv (accessed August 5, 2013).

3. Marco Bischof, "Humans Emit Biophotons—the Light of Our Cells," HeartSpring.net, January 30, 2011, http://heartspring.net/biophoton_meditation.html (accessed August 5, 2013).

4. Arthur M. Baker, "Raw Fresh Produce vs. Cooked Food," RawFoodHowTo.com, http://www.rawfoodhowto.com/raw-fresh-produce-vs-cooked.cfm (accessed August 5, 2013).

5. Timothy J. A. Key, Margaret Thorogood, Paul N. Appleby, and Michael L. Burr, "Dietary Habits and Mortality in 11,000 Vegetarians and Health Conscious People: Results of a 17-Year Follow

Up," *British Medial Journal* 313, no. 7060 (September 28, 1996): 775, http://www.bmj.com/content/313/7060/775 (accessed August 5, 2013).

6. PCC Sound Consumer, "Light Affects Nutrients," March 2012, http://www.pccnaturalmarkets.com/sc/1203/light_nutrients.html (accessed August 5, 2013).

7. Jon Ungoed-Thomas, "Official: Organic Really Is Better," *Sunday Times*, October 28, 2007, abstract viewed at http://www.timesonline.co.uk/tol/news/uk/health/article2753446.ece (accessed August 5, 2013).

8. J. D. Decuypere, "Radiation, Irradiation, and Our Food Supply," *The Decuypere Report*, http://www.healthalternatives2000.com/food-supply-report.html (accessed August 5, 2013).

9. US Food and Drug Administration, "Regulation of Foods Derived From Plants," statement of Lester M. Crawford before the Subcommittee on Conservation, Rural Development, and Research House Committee on Agriculture, June 17, 2003, http://www.fda.gov/NewsEvents/Testimony/ucm161037.htm (accessed August 5, 2013).

10. G. C. Smith, "Dietary Supplementation of Vitamin E to Cattle to Improve Shelf Life and Case Life of Beef for Domestic and International Markets," Colorado State University, referenced in EatWild.com, "Summary of Important Health Benefits of Grassfed Meats, Eggs, and Dairy," http://www.eatwild.com/healthbenefits.htm (accessed August 5, 2013).

11. World-wire.com, "American Public Health Association Supports Ban on Hormonal Milk and Meat," news release, November 13, 2009, http://www.world-wire.com/news/0911130001.html (accessed August 5, 2013).

12. Consumer Reports, "Chicken: Arsenic and Antibiotics," July 2007.

13. Tabitha Alterman, "Eggciting News!" MotherEarthNews.com, October 15, 2008, http://www.motherearthnews.com/Relish /Pastured-Eggs-Vitamin-D-Content.aspx (accessed August 5, 2013).

Chapter 5—Beverages, Fats, and Sweeteners— Choosing Healthy Accessories for Your Living Foods Diet

1. Joseph Mercola, "Aspartame's Hidden Dangers," Mercola.com, http://www.mercola.com/article/aspartame/hidden_dangers .htm (accessed October 7, 2013).

2. S. E. Swithers and T. L. Davidson, "A Role for Sweet Taste: Calorie Predictive Relations in Energy Regulation by Rats," *Behavioral Neuroscience* 122, no. 1 (February 2008): 161–173, referenced in ScienceDaily.com, "Artificial Sweeteners Linked to Weight Gain," February 11, 2008, http://www.sciencedaily.com/ releases/2008/02/080210183902.htm (accessed August 5, 2013).

3. WebMD.com, "Acai Berries and Acai Berry Juice—What Are the Health Benefits?", June 23, 2012, http://www.webmd.com/diet/ guide/acai-berries-and-acai-berry-juice-what-are-the-health -benefits (accessed August 5, 2013).

4. L. Scalfi, A. Coltorti, and F. Contaldo, "Postprandial Thermogenesis in Lean and Obese Subjects After Meals Supplemented With Medium-Chain and Long-Chain Triglycerides," *American Journal of Clinical Nutrition* 53, no. 5 (May 1, 1991): 1130–1133.

5. D. O. Ogbolu, A. A. Oni, O. A. Daini, and A. P. Oloko, "*In Vitro* Antimicrobial Properties of Coconut Oil on Candida Species in Ibadan, Nigeria," J*ournal of Medical Food* 10, no. 2 (June 2007): 384–387.

6. "Vegetable Oils/Fatty Acid Composition, Hexane Residues, Declaration, Pesticides (Organic Culinary Oils Only)," a joint campaign Basel city (specialist laboratory) and Basel county, http:// www.kantonslabor-bs.ch/files/berichte/Report0424.pdf (accessed August 5, 2013).

7. S. Couvreur, C. Hurtaud, C. Lopez, L. Delaby, and J. L. Peyraud, "The Linear Relationship Between the Proportion of Fresh Grass in the Cow Diet, Milk Fatty Acid Composition, and Butter Properties," *Journal of Dairy Science* 89, no. 6 (June 2006): 1956–1969, as referenced in EatWild.com, "Summary of Important Health Benefits of Grassfed Meats, Eggs, and Dairy."

8. S. O'Keefe, S. Gaskins-Wright, V. Wiley, and I-C. Chen, "Levels of Trans Geometrical Isomers of Essential Fatty Acids in Some Unhydrogenated U.S. Vegetable Oils," *Journal of Food Lipids* 1, no. 3 (September 1994): 165–176, referenced in WestonAPrice.org, "The Oiling of America," January 1, 2000, http://www.westonaprice.org/know-your-fats/525-the-oiling -of-america.html (accessed August 5, 2013).

9. *New York Times*, "Fat in Margarine Is Tied to Heart Problems," May 16, 1994, http://www.nytimes.com/1994/05/16/us/fat-in -margarine-is-tied-to-heart-problems.html (accessed October 13, 2013).

10. Alice Park, "Can Sugar Substitutes Make You Fat?" *Time*, February 10, 2008, http://www.time.com/time/health/ article/0,8599,1711763,00.html (accessed August 5, 2013).

11. Woodrow C. Monte, "Aspartame: Methanol and Public Health," *Journal of Applied Nutrition* 36, no. 1 (1984): 44, referenced in documentary *Sweet Misery* (Tucson, AZ: Sound and Fury Productions, 2004), http://www.soundandfury.tv/pages/sweet%20misery .html (accessed August 5, 2013); Dani Veracity, "The Link Between Aspartame and Brain Tumors: What the FDA Never Told You About Artificial Sweeteners," NaturalNews.com, September 22, 2005, http:// www.naturalnews.com/011804.html (accessed August 5, 2013).

Chapter 6—The Living Foods Meal Plan to Support Your Adrenal Glands

1. Decuypere, "Radiation, Irradiation, and Our Food Supply."

2. Lita Lee, "Microwaves and Microwave Ovens," May 14, 2001, http://www.litalee.com/documents/Microwaves%20And%20 Microwave%20Ovens.pdf (accessed August 6, 2013).

3. Decuypere, "Radiation, Irradiation, and Our Food Supply."

4. George J. Georgiou, "The Hidden Hazards of Microwave Cooking," *Journal for the American Association of Integrative Medicine* (online), April 2006, http://www.aaimedicine.com/jaaim/apr06/ hazards.php (accessed August 6, 2013).

5. Anthony Wayne and Lawrence Newell, "The Hidden Hazards of Microwave Cooking," Health-Science.com, http://www.health -science.com/microwave_hazards.html (accessed August 6, 2013).

Chapter 7—Best Tips for Making Fresh Juices and Smoothies

1. R. Akilen, A. Tsiami, D. Devendra, and N. Robinson, "Glycated Haemoglobin and Blood Pressure-Lowering Effect of Cinnamon in Multi-Ethnic Type 2 Diabetic Patients in the UK: A Randomized, Placebo-Controlled, Double-Blind Clinical Trial," *Diabetic Medicine* 27, no. 10 (October 2010): 1159–1167, http://onlinelibrary .wiley.com/doi/10.1111/j.1464-5491.2010.03079.x/full (accessed August 6, 2013).

2. Hong Wang, Guohua Cao, and Ronald L. Prior, "Total Antioxidant Capacity of Fruits," *Journal of Agricultural and Food Chemistry* 44, no. 3 (March 19, 1996): 701–705.

Chapter 8—Living Food, Juice, and Smoothie Recipes That Reduce Stress and Increase Positive Energy

1. Paul Bergner and Sharol Tilgner, "Gastrointestinal—Herbal Treatment for Ulcers," Medical Herbalism 3, no. 3: 1, 4–6, http:// www.medherb.com/Therapeutics/Gastrointestinal_-_Herbal_treat- ment_for_ulcers.htm (accessed August 6, 2013).

2. Jed W. Fahey et al., "Sulforaphane Inhibits Extracellular, Intracel- lular, and Antibiotic-Resistant Stomach Tumors," *Proceedings of the National Academy of Sciences* 99, no. 11 (May 28, 2002): 7610–7615.

FOR MORE INFORMATION

S IGN UP FOR the Juice Lady's free Juice Newsletter at www
.juiceladycherie.com.

Cherie's website

- www.juiceladycherie.com—information on juicing
  and weight loss

The Juice Lady's health and wellness juice retreats

I invite you to join us for a week that can change your life! Our
retreats offer gourmet organic raw foods with a three-day juice fast
midweek. We offer interesting, informative classes in a beautiful,
peaceful setting where you can experience healing and restoration
of body and soul. For more information, a brochure, and dates for
the retreats, call 866-843-8935.

Schedule a nutrition consultation with the Juice Lady

Call 866-843-8935.

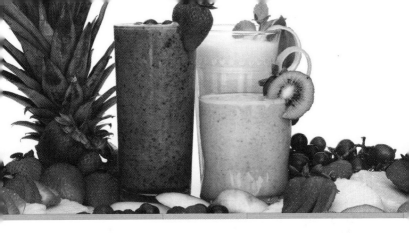

MORE BOOKS FROM THE JUICE LADY...

Jump-Start Your Diet and Lose Weight the Healthy Way

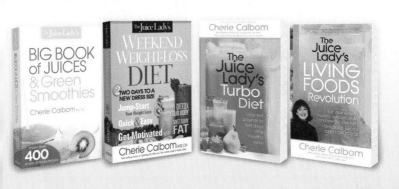

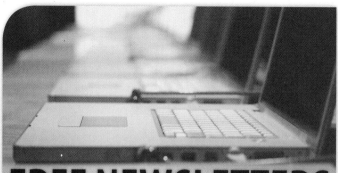
HILLSBORO PUBLIC LIBRARIES
Hillsboro, OR
Member of Washington County
COOPERATIVE LIBRARY SERVICES